Vision and Artifact

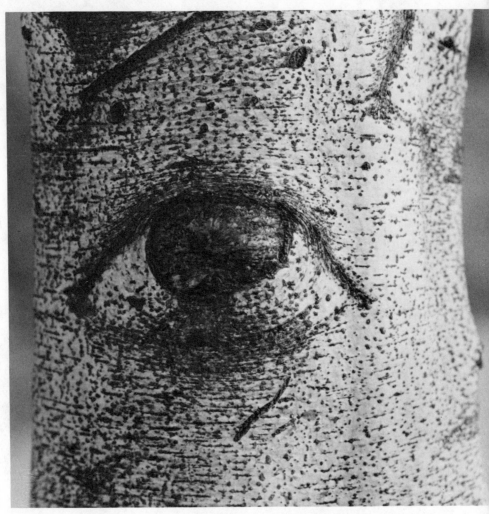

The Eye. Photo: Hannes Beckmann

12.95

VISION AND ARTIFACT

Mary Henle, Editor
Foreword by Rudolf Arnheim

Springer Publishing Company
New York

Springer Publishing Company, Inc.
200 Park Avenue South
New York, N.Y. 10003

76 77 78 79 80 / 10 9 8 7 6 5 4 3 2 1

Library of Congress Cataloging in Publication Data

Main entry under title:

Vision and artifact.

   CONTENTS: Visual perception: Held, R.
Single vision with doubled images. Metelli, F.
What does "more transparent" mean? Kanizsa, G.
and Gerbino, W. Convexity and symmetry in figure-
ground organization. [etc.]
   1. Visual perception—Addresses, essays, lectures.
2. Optical illusions—Addresses, essays, lectures.
3. Art—Psychology—Addresses, essays, lectures.
I. Henle, Mary, 1913 – II. Arnheim, Rudolf.
N71.V57   701'.15   76-3555
ISBN 0-8261-1960-3

Printed in the United States of America

Designed by Patrick Vitacco

To Rudolf Arnheim

Contents

Preface

On a lovely spring afternoon in 1974, in the charming garden of Gyorgy and Juliet Kepes in Cambridge, Massachusetts, a group of friends of Rudolf Arnheim met to celebrate his seventieth birthday. In friendship and in admiration of his contributions to his field and to theirs, they brought him their work and their good wishes. This unusual Festschrift consisted of scholarly papers side by side with graphic works; also included were letters and reminiscences. Quite in keeping with the scope of the man whose birthday they celebrated, the contributors represented the fields of art, art history, art criticism, mathematics, education, philosophy, and psychology. And, as an indication of his influence, papers arrived from three continents.

It is scarcely surprising that at the core of this variegated collection in honor of Rudolf Arnheim was a group of papers dealing with visual perception and visual art, for these terms may be considered a shorthand description of Arnheim's own major interests. These papers were selected for the present volume. But it was felt that a book on art and visual perception would not be complete without at least a note by Arnheim himself, and he kindly agreed to write a foreword.

Rudolf Arnheim has played a major role in shaping contemporary psychology of art. His work is the natural development of a lifelong immersion in the psychology of perception and thinking and in art, art criticism, and art history; he divided his time between laboratory studies and theoretical writings on the one hand and looking at art, talking about art, and thinking art, on the other. He was a student at the University of Berlin during the great days of its Psychological Institute, when Wolfgang Köhler, Max Wertheimer, and Kurt Lewin were developing the then young Gestalt psychology in one productive direction after another. The Gestalt psychology of perception differed from other approaches (then and largely now, too) in its emphasis on the whole properties and the expressiveness of perception, in understanding order as the outcome of dynamic processes, in its insistence that problems of value, of requiredness, could not be evaded by psychology. Productive thinking, too, was being studied in similar terms. Such a psychology was eminently suited for Arnheim's hybrid purposes.

Rudolf Arnheim is Professor Emeritus of the Psychology of Art at the Carpenter Center for the Visual Arts at Harvard University. A professorship in the psychology of art was an innovation for Harvard, for America, and, so far as I know, for the world. It would obviously not have been established had there not been a uniquely qualified candidate in the person of Professor Arnheim. Before assuming that newly created post, he taught the psychology of art and of expression, perception, and thinking at the Graduate Faculty of the New School for Social Research and at Sarah Lawrence College. His teaching was interrupted by two Guggenheim Fellowships, a Fulbright Lectureship in Japan, and by many invitations to lecture in America and abroad.

Among Arnheim's books, *Art and Visual Perception* (1954; new version, 1974) has long been the standard text for courses in the psychology of art, art appreciation, and the like. In 1956 *Film as Art* appeared; *Radio: An Art of Sound* was first published in 1936 and was republished in 1971. *Picasso's Guernica* (1962) is an essay in creativity; the artist's successive sketches are used to construct the biography of this painting. *Toward a Psychology of Art* (1966) is a collection of essays spanning a period of nearly twenty years and dealing with various aspects of Arnheim's favorite subjects: the sense of sight, the psychology of art, expression, artistic symbols, the creative process, art education. In 1969 *Visual Thinking* appeared, developing the bold thesis that "visual perception is visual thinking." *Entropy and Art* followed in 1971, an inquiry into order and disorder in nature and in art. Arnheim's influence is international, and his books have been translated into a number of languages.

The present volume will appeal to those many readers who have followed Arnheim's work and, indeed, to all those who are interested in art as it relates to visual perception and in perception as it bears on art. Artists, art theorists, art historians, psychologists, curators and museumgoers, professors and students will find here discussions of many of the questions they must have raised in their journeys into this frontier country between perception and art.

Boundaries not only separate, they also demarcate neighboring territories. Perceptual psychology has developed within the tradition of natural science, while art is classified among the humanities. The collection of essays, bridging perception and art, may thus be seen as a contribution to overcoming the science-humanism antinomy. Science as it illuminates art, problems of art as subjects for scientific analysis—these are the tacit themes of many of the essays in this volume.

It is a pleasure to acknowledge the special debt this book owes to its publisher. The unerring judgment, the sense of adventure, the sustaining good will of Ursula Springer have been essential conditions of shaping and completing it. And it is a special privilege to be associated with a volume in the spirit of the late Bernhard Springer.

Foreword

In Petronius' *Satyricon* the deplorable Trimalchio plays the host at a banquet distinguished by the luxurious variety of its dishes. In a speech of welcome he reviews the signs of the zodiac and comments that he himself was born under Cancer. "I was born under the Crab. So I have many legs to stand on, and many possessions by sea and land; for either one or the other suits your crab." Having been born under the same sign, I would observe first that the many possessions do not necessarily follow and second, that to stand on many legs, as I have done in my own professional interests for a lifetime, is rewarding but tricky. Especially, however, I would stress still another property of the crab that Trimalchio neglected—namely that of walking sideways. The traffic problem this creates is obvious, considering that everybody else proceeds forward to his defined goal. Making the best of it, I have found that to cross the paths of so many pioneers has enriched my own thinking immeasurably, and if the contributors to this volume have anything in common besides their persistent interest in vision it is that they do not seem to have minded when I waylaid them now and then.

In fact, these psychologists, philosophers, historians, educators, and critics have been productively curious about what is going on to their right and left, and all of them harbor some sort of overview of what the field of vision amounts to as a whole. Inevitably such an overview looks like a network of approaches, for although the world of reality hangs together seamlessly and is ultimately indivisible, our inroads remain particular and linear and add up to a map rather than to the universe. If nevertheless we would sit together and try to sketch a model of our subject in its principal ranges, something like the following might emerge.

Human eyes are only small objects, each barely the size of a wrist watch. But it is in the nature of things that while their func- xiii tion and performance may be simple, the mechanisms that let them do it are admirably intricate. The ways in which the eyes and the adjoining sections of the nervous system receive and transduce light, reconstruct shape, and make color vision possible have led to discoveries of which the present volume contains some striking examples.

Vision is not a physical object like the eye but a mental experience, and the discrepancy between the smallness of the organ and the immensity of the expanse covered by vision has been a puzzle since antiquity. Visual experience is the principal gatherer of knowledge because it offers the best bridge between consciousness and the world of the body. Its study, therefore, involves basic ontological problems and must be called a branch of epistemology. The physical world appears visually only in translation, and the result of any translation depends on the properties of the medium. In our case, the medium consists first of all of the optical system of image formation. The ingenious ways in which the bias of the projective image is compensated for by processes in the retina and the brain are described in the many studies that can be grouped under the heading of psychophysics because they compare the physical stimulus with the mental effect. Such studies, for example, explore the conditions that prevent misleading retinal motions from being reflected in consciousness or provide for the emergence of sensible boundaries where none exist in the external world; they formulate the particular circumstances that create transparency from opaque materials, and so forth.

When visual phenomena are reasonably simple they can be measured and counted. This is true particularly for the controlled conditions of laboratory experiments. What is seen in the outside world is generally more complex, not only because the perceived objects and events themselves are rarely limited to simple shapes but also because the viewer's reception is modified by a full load of past experience, expectation, understanding, and need. Under such conditions, quantitative measurements of the resulting experience are rarely possible and often inappropriate. What can sometimes be done, however, is to take measurements of the physical pattern that gives rise to the percept—for example, to establish the numerical proportions of a building or painting. Here the scientist and the artist can join forces. In fact, the alliance of intuitive insight, which is the principal guide of the artist, with the intellectual analysis cultivated by the scientist offers the most promising approach to our understanding of visual phenomena.

It is not sufficient to speak of the relation between the physical world and the percepts derived from that world as though it were a mere difference. More and more we come to appreciate the gathering of sensory information as a creative process. The retinal input is given intelligible form in keeping with the properties of the stimuli on the one hand and those of the processing medium on the other. The capacities of the medium grow, as the mind grows, from the grasping of the simplest shapes and relations to more and more complex ones. And corresponding to this development, the complexity of the patterns invented by man for his use increases with age. This is strikingly reflected in the stages observable in the art work of children and early periods of culture.

Art is also a telling illustration of the fact that vision has a fundamental impact on the physical world. Painting and sculpture exist only because there are eyes by which to make and receive them. What we call architecture, as distinguished from the mere building of shelters, is almost totally visual. And even in the biological world the eye's ability to observe the presence and behavior of things has remained, shall we say, not unnoticed. The influence of vision on the shapes and colors of plants and animals for protection and advertising is well known.

But it is only in the interest of tidy concepts that we distinguish between features which exist for the sake of vision alone and others whose visual aspects are only reflections of quite different functions fulfilled by shapes in what one might call the transvisual world. The works of architecture and technology, executed by artists, engineers, spiders, or bees, enrich the aesthetic sense by a coincidence of physical function and beautifully organized appearance. At the same time, visual images would be of little value to us if they were not the carriers of messages about things that are not visual.

Here we touch upon the humanly most precious power of vision, namely that of endowing thought with the form of perceptual symbols. Although vision reports only about the outer surface of things, it uses the inherent expression of shape, color, and movement to make philosophical, religious, and social statements visually intelligible.

In my own terms I have tried to describe here a model of the world of vision as it might emerge if the contributors to the present collection of articles were to sit together and discuss the matter. However, in the mind of each of these men and women the subject would assume an appearance all of its own, and it is the variety of approaches derived from the different backgrounds of the authors that makes this book on vision unique. To have been the *causa transiens* of this picturesque meeting of minds is a great satisfaction to me, especially since it reflects so accurately my own aspirations and so gratifyingly goes beyond what I have tried to do.

Experts from different disciplines are not easily brought together for a common purpose, and it would not have happened this time without the laborious efforts of the editor. Not unexpectedly, Mary Henle is still another Crab, one who has used the opportunities of her constellation not only to traverse broad areas of psychology, philosophy, and history in her own work but also to create and cultivate those human links between explorers and thinkers that are a necessary condition for any synthesis of thought. How a person can do so much for others while being so productive on her own remains Mary Henle's secret. All I can do here is to thank her on behalf of her many debtors and in the name of the one person for whom I can speak with some authority.

Rudolf Arnheim

Contributors

Rudolf Arnheim, Ph.D. Professor of the psychology of art, emeritus, Harvard University

Dore Ashton, M.A. Professor of art history, The Cooper Union

Howard Gardner, Ph.D. Research associate, Boston Veterans Administration Hospital and Boston University School of Medicine; Co-Director, Project Zero, Harvard University

James J. Gibson, Ph.D. Professor of psychology emeritus and professor, Graduate Faculty, Cornell University

Richard Held, Ph.D. Professor of experimental psychology, Massachusetts Institute of Technology

Walter Hess, Ph.D. Professor of the history of art, Hochschule für bildende Künste, Berlin

Leo M. Hurvich, Ph.D. Professor of psychology, University of Pennsylvania

Dorothea Jameson University professor of psychology and visual science, University of Pennsylvania; adjunct professor of psychology, Columbia University

Gaetano Kanizsa, Ph.D. Professor of psychology, University of Trieste

John M. Kennedy, Ph.D. Professor of psychology, Scarborough College, University of Toronto

Fabio Metelli, Ph.D. Professor of psychology, University of Padua

Ernest Nash Late founder and director of the Fototeca, American Academy, Rome

Henry Schaefer-Simmern, H.L.D. Professor of art, St. Mary's College of California, Moraga, California

Eduard F. Sekler, Ph.D. Professor of architecture, Osgood Hooker Professor of Visual Arts, and director of the Carpenter Center for the Visual Arts, Harvard University

Marianne L. Teuber, M.A. Art historian, Arlington, Massachusetts

Hans Wallach, Ph.D. Professor of psychology, Swarthmore College

Wolfgang M. Zucker, Ph.D. Henry Peterson Professor of Philosophy, Upsala College, East Orange, New Jersey

I

VISUAL PERCEPTION

This part deals with a number of the special problems of perception that the artist often has to solve technically, the psychologist experimentally and theoretically. It is obvious that many perceptual problems enter into the work of the artist other than those included here. But the examples in this part are sufficient to illustrate an important relation between art and the psychology of perception. Art is a testing ground for theories of perception; these theories can often illuminate specific aspects of the work of art and place them in a more general context.

How is it that human beings, equipped with two eyes, see a single world (or a single picture)? The history of this fascinating problem from ancient times to the present is discussed by Held.

Perceptual transparency is often created by artists who have only opaque materials at their disposal. Metelli examines experimentally the conditions of such transparency; his investigation raises new problems as to the nature of transparency.

Art (as well as perception under almost all conditions) has to deal with the organization of the visual field into figure and background. That the factors governing this organization have heretofore been incompletely investigated is shown by Kanizsa and Gerbino. They demonstrate the role of convexity in figure-ground organization and point to further problems for study.

Another fascinating aspect of certain visual displays is the appearance of contours under conditions of homogeneous stimulation—i.e., under conditions where no physical correlate of the contour is present. Such contours are investigated by Kennedy, who relates them to pictorial perception.

Jameson and Hurvich discuss the physiological processes responsible for brightness constancy, contrast, and assimilation in perception. They find compelling illustrations of these effects in works of art.

Why does the painted head of a portrait seem to follow us as   3 we walk past the picture in a gallery? This is the question Wallach raises. He relates this phenomenon to recent perceptual investigations of why our perceived three-dimensional world remains stable, despite retinal displacements, when we move about in it.

A final paper in this section is of obvious relevance to the making and viewing of films. Gibson and his co-workers ask how, when an object disappears from the visual field, we know whether it ceases to exist or simply drops out of sight. In a number of cases they are able to specify the stimulus information that enables observers to distinguish between permanent and impermanent parts of the environment.

Richard Held

Single Vision with Doubled Images: An Historic Problem

How does the observer gain unitary vision of the world of objects despite the doubling of images formed on the two eyes? The question was raised in ancient times and recurs in a qualified way even in our time. The problem begins with the belief that the perception of an object entails some sort of representation of it in mind (we shall call it the *effigy*) which is identified with the workings of the sensory mechanisms and their connections with more central parts of the observer's nervous system (Held, 1965). The mind is informed of properties of the object through the senses, and, if the information is to be accurate and useful, it must be correctly conveyed to the locus of the effigy. Accordingly, ancient commentators asserted that objects cast off replicas of themselves which were conveyed to the senses and thence to the seat of perception. With increasing knowledge of the physical media of conveyance and of the anatomy and physiology of sensory mechanisms, this simple notion could not be maintained. However, the demand that the effigy resemble its object and, consequently, that representations adequate for this purpose be conveyed to the center of perception, was retained as a kind of prescription—I shall call it a *metatheory*—to be fulfilled by any adequate psychological theory of perception. And, by implication, any attempt to supply a physiological model, assumed to correlate with the psychological process, must also obey this prescription.

The problem of the two eyes is, of course, a special aspect of the general metatheory demanding semblance in the effigy. Clearly, if there is a doubling of what is transmitted from the object to the eyes, there must be a corresponding process of unification to satisfy the demand of the ancient logic. The doubled image must somehow be resolved into a single coherent effigy by action of the visual system. This demand for unification of the two images of the single object is then part of the 5

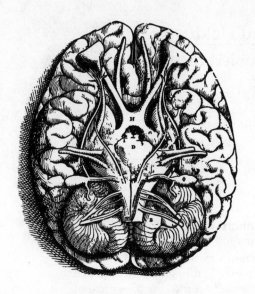

1 Woodcut showing the human brain viewed from below and showing retina at I, optic chiasm at H, and continuation of optic nerves at G. From Andreas Vesalius' *De Humani Corporis Fabrica*, Basel, 1543.

metatheory of perception we have mentioned above, and we shall briefly examine some of its historical vicissitudes.

The second-century anatomist Galen was apparently one of the first to consider seriously the importance of the anatomy of the eye and optic nerves for questions of vision and thereby to lay a foundation for the development of models satisfying the metatheory (Polyak, 1957). He identified the lens of the eye as the part sensitive to the impressions from outside and considered the optic nerves as hollow tubes joined at the optic chiasm and carrying a fluid. The gross features of the anatomy of the visual system are shown in Figure 1. One of the functions Galen assigned to the chiasm was the uniting of the impressions made on the two eyes, although he was not very specific as to how this was accomplished (Polyak, 1957; Ronchi, 1956).

The first known attempt to resolve the problem by a detailed model was that of Alhazen, the eleventh-century Arab physician, who has been called the creator of physiological optics (Ronchi, 1956). Alhazen's theory of image formation described a point-to-point projection of object-to-image points on the anterior surface of the lens which preserved the identity of form and orientation of image with respect to object. He developed this ingenious, but erroneous, theory of image formation partly because of his unwillingness to accept an inverted and reverted retinal image. Since Alhazen identified the orientation of the image with that of the perception of the originating object, the inverted image would yield a false perception. The metatheory which demanded semblance between image and percept thus

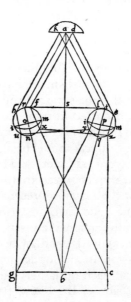

2   Diagram of object *gbc* casting images *hrf* and *lte* on retinae of the two eyes which, in turn, are projected to *kad* at optic chiasm. Attributed to Alhazen by Vitellio in his *Perspectiva*, 1572.

may have delayed an advance in the science of optics until the time of Kepler, five centuries later.

Clearly, in the case of the two images formed in separate eyes, the problem of unification was not optical in nature; it had to be resolved by consideration of the structure and function of the nervous system with which the eyes communicated. Just as the general metatheory demanding preservation of similarity of form and orientation helped determine Alhazen's model of image formation, so the related metatheory demanding unification of the two images to gain the single percept of the object influenced his model of function of the optic nerves posterior to the eyeballs. In accord with this demand, Alhazen first concluded that vision could not be completed in the eye. Instead, the eyes were instruments aiding the conveyance of representations to the place where they could be unified. Following Galen's lead, Alhazen chose the optic chiasm as the first and most obvious place for unification of the images (ten Doesschate, 1962). He had claimed that the posterior surface of the lens refracted the rays, which had formed an image on the anterior surface and then penetrated the lens so as to allow them to continue through the course of the optic nerve. At the chiasm Alhazen depicted a point-by-point superimposition of the points coming from the two images formed on the lens (see Fig. 2, taken from Vitellio, 1572). This model of conveyance through the nerves and of point-by-point projection onto the chiasm now satisfied the demand for unification of the two images made so much more sophisticated by Alhazen's analysis of

Richard Held

7

image formation. Note that the model accomplishes its task by the simple formalism of having the rays traveling from the lenses to the chiasm go through the inverse of the transformation that occurred in projection from object to eyes. The model of neural function is then a precise, although inverted, counterpart of his optical model of light transmission. As we shall see, this stratagem was later used by Descartes for a similar purpose.

Alhazen recognized that the chiasm was not the final destination of the visual representation. The meaning of the extension of the optic tract, posterior to the chiasm, to the main mass of the brain remained an issue. In the thirteenth century, Roger Bacon, heavily dependent upon Alhazen's account, discussed transmission in the optic nerves in the following terms. He stated that each optic nerve extends from the eye to enter the opposite side of the brain, passing through the chiasm on its way. He reasoned that if there were not this crossing of the nerves, the extension of the optic nerve from chiasm to brain on the same side would require transmission through a fairly sharp angle with apex at the chiasm (see Fig. 1). "But this would hinder vision, because vision always selects straight lines as far as possible" (Bacon, 1928). Clearly, Bacon's model of transmission in the nerves was analogous to that of light, although elsewhere he does suggest that the properties of nerve make possible some modification of the supposed propagation in straight lines. He also appears to suggest that—apart from whatever unification of the two representations may occur at the chiasm—the paths of transmission from eye to brain are completely crossed. The course of transmission through the chiasm becomes a considerable issue in later centuries, as we shall see.

We can next consider Descartes' model of vision (see Fig. 3) published in his *Traité de l'Homme* in 1686. Many decades prior to the publication of this schema, Kepler had advanced the essentially correct geometrical theory of image formation by a lens accepting the implied inversion and reversion of the retinal images cast by external objects (Crombie, 1964). Accordingly, Descartes shows the optics of the two eyes inverting the images on the retinae. But the nervous system behind the retina is depicted as re-inverting and unifying the internal representation by point-to-point projections to the pineal gland. The stratagem of reproducing a replica of the object by having the visual system perform a transformation inverse to that of the optical one is, in principle, the same as that employed by Alhazen. The choice of a site of unification deeper in the brain was undoubtedly dictated by Des-

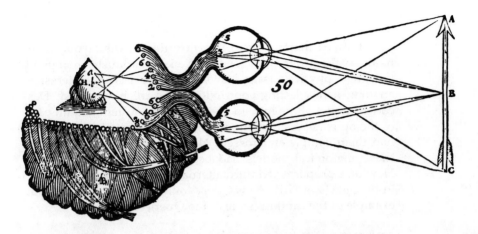

3 Object *abc* casts images *531* on both retinae, which are, in turn, projected to positions *abc* on pineal gland. Diagram from Descartes' *Traité de l'Homme*, 1686.

cartes' thoroughgoing adherence to the body-machine doctrine. But his choice of a single midline structure—the pineal body—has the same logic as Alhazen's choice of the chiasm. Such a structure offers the simplest locus for superimposition by point-to-point projection of the images common to the two eyes.

The mechanism employed by Descartes to achieve the internal transformation has one other interesting aspect from our point of view. Unlike Roger Bacon, Descartes had no qualms about extending each of the optic nerves from the eye to the brain on the same side, despite the large bend at what is presumably the location of the chiasm. Clearly, his model of transmission in the nervous system is no longer analogous to that of light. It is mechanical, and, although unconstrained by the requirement of transmission in straight lines, it does limit transmission to separate conducting pathways in order to maintain point-to-point projection. Thus we can note that although the physical model of image formation by the lens and the speculative model of transmission in the nervous system have both been changed, the combination satisfies the unaltered metatheory. Descartes ingeniously managed to make the internal effigy copy the external object.

We may note parenthetically that when, and to the extent that, the object-effigy resemblance is questioned, a metaphysical problem arises if knowledge of the world has been made dependent upon the relation. The intricate bearing of optics on this issue has often been noted (Graham, 1929).

Richard
Held

9

The next major step in interpretation of the layout of the neural pathways from the eyes was taken, curiously enough, by the great physicist Isaac Newton, whose passing interest in anatomy left a lasting contribution. As we have noted, Descartes' model of the human visual nervous system had no parts of the optic nerves crossing the midline; Bacon, by implication, had them completely crossed. No general preference between these anatomical models had been established at the time of Newton's proposal of a third alternative (published as Query 15 in his *Opticks* of 1704). This Query, only a paragraph long, is an example of the cautious style of the Queries.

Are not the Species of Objects seen with both Eyes united where the optick Nerves meet before they come into the Brain, the Fibres on the right side of both Nerves uniting there, and after union going thence into the Brain in the Nerve which is on the right side of the Head, and the Fibres on the left side of both Nerves uniting in the same place, and after union going into the Brain in the Nerve which is on the left side of the Head, and these two Nerves meeting in the Brain in such a manner that their Fibres make but one entire Species of Picture, half of which on the right side of the Sensorium comes from the right side of both Eyes through the right side of both optick Nerves to the place where the Nerves meet, and from thence on the right side of the Head into the Brain, and the other half on the left side of the Sensorium comes in like manner from the left side of both Eyes. For the optick Nerves of such Animals as look the same way with both Eyes (as of Men, Dogs, Sheep, Oxen, etc.) meet before they come into the Brain, but the optick Nerves of such Animals as do not look the same way with both Eyes (as of Fishes, and of the Chameleon) do not meet, if I am rightly inform'd.

Newton was convinced, unlike Descartes, that the seat of sentience was not located in a single structure situated on the midline of the brain. Instead, the Sensorium was represented bilaterally in the two halves of the brain. He based his argument for partial decussation of the optic nerves on the observation that animals having lateral eyes with little or no overlap of their fields of vision—fish, for example—have optic nerves that remain separated and cross each other at the chiasm; whereas those that have overlapping visual fields have these nerves joined at the chiasm. The reason for the difference, asserted Newton, must then be superimposition of the overlapping parts of the fields, as centrally projected, to eliminate doubling of the internal representation. This can be achieved most simply by combination of the half fields of each eye (as in Fig. 4).

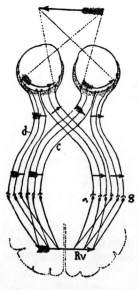

4 From S. Ramon y Cajal, *Recollections of My Life.* Cambridge: M.I.T. Press, 1966.

Newton's model of partial crossing of the optic nerves was proven correct much later by studies of the fine structure of the chiasmal fibers; consequently, he is credited with the discovery of the partial decussation of optic nerve fibers in the chiasm. In the absence of any evidence that the then contemporary anatomists believed in the hemidecussation suggested by Newton, one must conclude that this anatomical discovery was the result of the application of a model of connection satisfying the perceptual metatheory that the neural substrate for the perception of a single object would not allow for a doubled representation. Thus this metatheory of perception apparently led to a deduction about anatomy that happened to be correct. Here is one of the rare cases in which the application of a psychological metatheory not only influenced the progress of another science but actually guided a discovery.

We may also note that Newton was not concerned with maintaining the orientation of the internal representation similar to that of the object it represents as were Descartes and previous commentators. Projection of the right and left hemiretinae to the same sides of the brain necessarily implies reversal of the representations of left and right parts of the visual fields in the brain (see Fig. 4). Thus, although Newton applied the metatheory of the unified representation, he discarded the demand for an effigy having the same spatial orientation as its objects. A few years later, Berkeley advanced his critical analysis of the problem of the inverted image (1709).

Another significant new departure was Newton's use of

Richard
Held

11

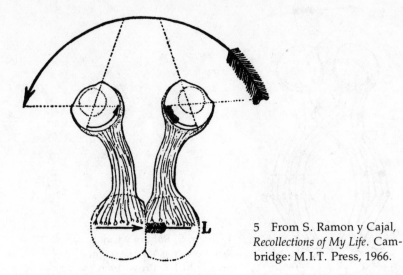

5 From S. Ramon y Cajal, *Recollections of My Life*. Cambridge: M.I.T. Press, 1966.

comparative morphology—namely, his comparison between species of animals having separate fields of vision for the two eyes (panoramic vision) with those having overlapping fields of vision. In taking this comparative approach, Newton differed greatly from Descartes, for whom such comparison was presumably precluded by the assumption that animals lack sensibility. Newton may have been influenced in this approach by the contemporary English interest in classification of species, as represented especially by John Ray, its ablest exponent (Nordenskiöld, 1928).

Newton's interpretation of the anatomy of the chiasm continued to have its critics until the turn of this century, when the anatomist Santiago Ramon y Cajal once again took up the question of the chiasm. By this time the topographical representation of the retina on the cerebral cortex was fairly well established (Polyak, 1957). Much evidence pointed to the validity of earlier speculations on a point-to-point (region-to-region would be more accurate) projection from retina to cerebral cortex. Although this projection entailed considerable geometrical distortion, the topography of the retina appeared to be preserved.

Cajal's initial motive for reconsidering the anatomy of the chiasm was a renewed claim, supported by at least one eminent contemporary anatomist (Kölliker), that the fibers of the human optic nerves were completely crossed at the chiasm. Although thoroughly convinced of his own anatomical evidence for a noncrossing pathway, Cajal also wrote that the partial decussation, originally proposed by Newton, was " . . . an unavoidable

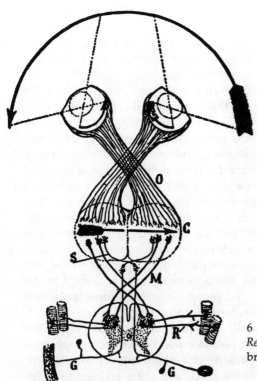

6 From S. Ramon y Cajal, *Recollections of My Life*. Cambridge: M.I.T. Press, 1966.

physiological postulate, . . ." without which we "would have been unable . . . to explain how we perceive only one visual image when the brain receives two almost identical" (Ramon y Cajal, 1966). Having so termed Newton's discovery, Cajal raised the deeper question of the reason for decussation of the optic nerves, whether partial or complete. "Hence, in order that the mental perception may be unified and may agree exactly with the external reality, or in other words, in order that the image conveyed through the right eye may be continuous with that conveyed through the left eye, the intercrossing of the optic paths from side to side is quite necessary; a total crossing in animals with panoramic vision, a partial crossing in animals endowed with a common visual field." His interpretation took the form of first showing how, if the nerves of a creature with lateral-seeing eyes were not crossed, the right and left halves of the environment would be reversed with a resulting discontinuity of the central projections of the two fields (Fig. 5). Crossing the nerves restores the continuity of the fields (Fig. 6). The partial decussation of the mammalian chiasm is then simply an extension of his rule for maintaining continuity plus Newton's method of maintaining the single central representation (Fig.4).

Richard Held

13

In contrast to Newton's use of the perceptual metatheory to make a discovery, Cajal used the metatheory to justify the functional significance of his anatomical findings.

Cajal's Figure 6 shows motor pathways connected to the optic lobes. Anticipations of these completed reflex paths are to be found in earlier commentators (Descartes, 1686; Newton, 1704) but Cajal brings in a new consideration. He cautiously suggests that the decussations found in both motor and other sensory pathways may have been brought about as a result of the original visual decussation, presumably in the course of evolution. He gives no further explanation of why decussation in the visual system should produce decussation in motor and somatic sensory systems. But we may hazard the guess that Cajal had in mind the matching, by re-reversion, of left and right halves of visual space with their counterparts in motor and somatic space. Implicit in this argument is a resolution of the problem of the reverted (and inverted) internal representations by reference now to movement and to intersensory agreement. This resolution is essentially that proposed by Berkeley (1709) but now given an explicit neural embodiment. Although perceived continuity is identified with continuity of neural representation, perception of the orientation of a visible object (as Cajal terms it) is no more to be identified with that of its representation in the brain than it is with the image on the retina.

After Cajal, neither the anatomy of the chiasm nor the superposition of the central representations of the two retinae were any longer a matter for serious debate, but the question of the continuity of the central projections of right and left half fields broken by the midline of the brain remained. Let me mention several modern instances of this concern. In their theory of figural aftereffects, Wolfgang Köhler and Hans Wallach correlate distance between visible positions with the inverse of the density of a hypothetical current between the two corresponding positions in the visual cortex (Köhler & Wallach, 1944). To account for the obvious continuity (zero distance) across the two lateral half fields of vision, they suggest that the interhemispheric connection (the great fiber bundle formed by the corpus callosum) is of very slight resistance to the passage of the hypothetical currents. Consequently, it can serve to bring together and preserve the continuity of the two halves of the visual field. Here, Köhler used a model drawn directly from physics to satisfy an aspect of the traditional metatheory.

Köhler's model was criticized for paying too little attention to the fine structure of the brain. And, indeed, within a decade or two of its proposal, evidence was obtained for neural connections through the corpus callosum which could be held responsible for the continuity of the two half fields of vision. Recently, Hubel and Wiesel reported evidence that callosal nerve fibers link cortical cells whose receptive fields span the vertical meridian, hence providing connections across the half fields (Hubel & Wiesel, 1967). Interestingly enough, they prefaced their paper with the following statement: "The fact that our visual fields appear uniform, with no obvious interruption along the vertical midline, would seem to call for connections linking the two hemispheres." The authors do not further elaborate on this point. Presumably they believe that continuity of a contour anywhere in the visual field is achieved as a result of connections among cells representing adjacent segments of the contour. Consequently, in order to achieve this connectivity across the midline, connections must be made across the hemispheres and the large commissural fiber tracts are most likely to contain such pathways. Berlucchi and Rizzolatti, two other contemporary investigators of the same neural system, prefaced their report with a slightly more explicit statement: "Perceptual unity of the cerebral hemispheres in the act of seeing is thought to result largely from the activity of commissural pathways, especially the corpus callosum" (Berlucchi & Rizzolatti, 1968).

With the discovery of evidence for connections across the midline, one might suppose that a complete model of the visual system was available which satisfied the metatheoretical demands as well as could be expected. The central projections of the retinae are superimposed in the appropriate order with connections across the only substantial break in topography—namely, the midline. However, several sets of recent observations raise new questions about this conception.

First of all, detailed studies of the vision of people suffering agenesis of the corpus callosum and certain other midline structures reveal no abnormalities of the type that are suggested by the traditional interpretation (Sperry, 1968). Despite the absence of corpus callosum and other telencephalic commissures, no break in the continuity of the visual field across the vertical midline has been noted. There remain connections across the midline through the midbrain commissures, but these must be several synapses in length and, hence, quite different from transcortical connections within the cerebrum. This evidence makes one doubt that connections known and inferred to exist within the cerebrum are in fact responsible for perceived continuity.

A second set of observations which raises a problem is that

Richard
Held

which, in recent years, has demonstrated the existence of not one retinotopic projection in the cerebral cortex but two, three, and perhaps four (Bilge et al., 1967). The initial discoveries of the fine structure of the visual nervous system made it appear that the system was carefully designed to produce a unitary neural representation from the two retinal images. The discovery of multiple representations appears to contradict this conclusion and leaves us wondering about their functions.

New knowledge of the visual nervous system, gained by studies of the electrical responses of single cells, leads one to suspect that the primary function of the superposition of the topographic projections of the two eyes is stereopsis (Barlow et al., 1967). The extreme precision of stereoscopic acuity would, it would appear, only be made possible by bringing together the information from corresponding local areas of the two retinae. Evidence bearing on the detailed neural connections of the visual cortex indicates that the nervous structures at this level are primarily designed for analysis of local spatial features of visual stimulation on the retina (Hubel & Wiesel, 1962). This evidence, in turn, suggests that continuity of contour across large distances on the retina is probably not a consequence of short (monosynaptic) connections between adjacent regions of cortex. According to this reasoning, the layouts of the topographic projections from retina to cortex are not to be regarded as representing a distorted metric of the perceived distribution of contours and forms. Speaking metaphorically, these maps are not directly read as one would read a geographic map. Rather, the information recorded at sites on the map encodes local characteristics of regions of the image on the retina and, hence, the visual scene. Global properties, such as continuity of long contours, are presumably extracted by analysis of combinations of local features. The metrical properties of visual space may be established by similar means (Held, 1968). In any event, spatial properties of the percept can no longer be identified with those of the topography of the cortical projections. Consequently, the unity of the perceived world is not discrepant with a multiplicity of internal representations whether they originate in the two eyes or otherwise. The mode of representation of space must be considerably more abstract; to this extent at least, a reformulation of the ancient metatheory is required.

The vicissitudes of the problem that has been reviewed show that the influence of models from the several sciences that we have discussed has not been a one-way affair but rather an interaction. Metatheories have determined the use of these models and such models have in turn influenced the demands made by the metatheory. If the logic of this interaction has any generality, it would appear that models from nonpsychological disciplines have served as parts of theories of psychology when they have satisfied the demands and constraints of relevant metatheories.

A metatheory is an explicit or implicit formulation of what a process must accomplish; it is a directive for theorizing and model building. Proponents of metatheories are often aware that the actual mode of operation of the system being dealt with will only be established when an adequate model of the system is at hand. Models are imported from other sciences with varying degrees of success. Their use has run the gamut from claims of being literally embodied within the system being described to milder claims that the system behaves as if it were working according to the operation of the model. Most frequently, these models have been applied only to be discarded later as the result either of new knowledge inconsistent with the old model or of the availability of a more convincing model for dealing with the same knowledge.

When, as has occasionally been the case, such a model is actually shown to be embodied in the system, it ceases to be part of psychology as such. Thus the advent of Kepler's theory of image formation by a lens once and for all removed the problem of the formation of the retinal image from the purview of what we now call psychology and clearly established it as part of physics (Crombie, 1964). Another clear example of this sort of evolution of theory comes from the history of color vision. A century and a half elapsed between the speculations of Thomas Young concerning three types of retinal units differing in sensitivity to hues (1802) and the recent discoveries by Wald and others of three photopigments in the retina having different spectral sensitivities (1964). If this sort of development of theory were inevitable, psychological processes would always be reducible to the workings of the nervous system. And a conviction that such a reduction is in fact inevitable has, of course, created disbelief in some quarters in the possibility of an independent science of psychology. But such inevitability is far from obvious in principle and very far from achievement in fact.

Psychologists will, no doubt, continue to be influenced by models from other sciences which fit their metatheoretical prejudices. In doing so, I suspect that they follow a tradition shared by investigators of many other disciplines.

Richard
Held

17

REFERENCES   Bacon, R. *Opus majus*. Philadelphia: University of Pennsylvania Press, 1928.

Barlow, H.B., Blakemore, C., & Pettigrew, J.D. The neural mechanism of binocular depth discrimination. *Journal of Physiology 193* (1967): 327–342.

Berkeley, G. *An essay towards a new theory of vision*. 1709.

Berlucchi, G., & Rizzolatti, G. Binocularly driven neurons in visual cortex of split-chiasm cats. *Science 159* (1968): 308–310.

Bilge, M., Bingle, A., Seneviratne, K.N., & Whitteridge, D. A map of the visual cortex in the cat. *Journal of Physiology 191* (1967): 116–118.

Crombie, A.C. Kepler: De modo visionis. In: *Mélanges Alexandre Koyré*, Vol. 1. Paris: Hermann, 1964.

Descartes, R. *Traité de l'homme*. 1686.

Graham, E. *Optics and vision*. Doctoral Dissertation, Columbia University, 1929.

Held, R. Object and effigy. In: *Structure in art and in science*. G. Kepes (Ed.). New York: Braziller, 1965.

Held, R. Dissociation of visual functions by deprivation and re-arrangement. *Psychologische Forschung 31* (1968): 338–348.

Hubel, D., & Wiesel, T. Receptive fields, binocular interaction, and functional architecture in the cat's visual cortex. *Journal of Physiology 106* (1962): 106–153.

Hubel, D., & Wiesel, T. Cortical and callosal connections concerned with the vertical meridian of visual fields in the cat. *Journal of Neurophysiology 30* (1967): 1561–1573.

Köhler, W., & Wallach, H. Figural after-effects: An investigation of visual processes. *Proceedings of the American Philosophical Society 88* (1944): 269–357.

Newton, I. *Opticks*. 1704.

Nordenskiöld, E. *The history of biology*. New York: Tudor, 1928.

Polyak, S. *The vertebrate visual system*. Chicago: University of Chicago Press, 1957.

Ramon y Cajal, S. *Recollections of my life*. Cambridge, Mass.: M.I.T. Press, 1966.

Ronchi, V. *Histoire de la lumière*. Paris: Librairie Armand Colin, 1956.

Sperry, W. Mental unity following surgical disconnection of the cerebral hemispheres. In: *The Harvey Lecture Series*, Vol. 62. New York: Academic Press, Inc., 1968.

ten Doesschate, G. Oxford and the revival of optics in the thirteenth century. *Vision Research 1* (1962) 313–342.

Vesalius, A. *De humani corporis fabrica*. Basel, 1543.

Vitellio. *Perspectiva*. 1572.

Wald, G. The receptors of human color vision. *Science 145* (1964): 1007–1017.

Young, T. On the theory of light and colours. *Philosophical Transactions of the Royal Society of London 92* (1802): 18–21.

Fabio Metelli

What Does "More Transparent" Mean?
A Paradox

The perception of transparency may be studied for different purposes, but the main one seems to be to describe the phenomenal aspects of transparency and to discover the conditions that give rise to them. When possible, laws that allow predictions about the phenomenon ought to be formulated.

First of all, the conditions of the phenomenon have to be specified. Thus it becomes clear that, contrary to what seems self-evident, physical transparency is neither a necessary nor a sufficient condition for the perception of transparency; therefore a more precise and restrictive definition of perceptual transparency is needed. Physical transparency is present everywhere, as we always see objects through the (physically) transparent air. But under these conditions we do not perceive transparency. We perceive transparency only when the transparent object or layer is perceived, in addition to the objects seen through it (Metelli, 1974a, p.91).

We commonly speak of more or less transparent objects. The present discussion will be restricted to achromatic colors. (My current research has been confined to achromatic colors to avoid excessive complexity of conditions.) If we use various nonselective filters to cover a given black and white figure, we perceive various degrees of transparency, and transparency decreases as the density of the filters increases. The same result can be obtained without having recourse to physical transparency. By the use of different shades of gray cardboard (Metzger, 1953, pp. 127–131), figures can be constructed which give rise to a clear impression of transparency (Figs. 1, 2). With variation of the difference between the grays forming the central square, which is perceived as transparent, the degree of perceived transparency varies. The more similar the shades of gray in the central region, the greater the perceived opacity, and therefore the less the transparency of the square. (See appendix.)

19

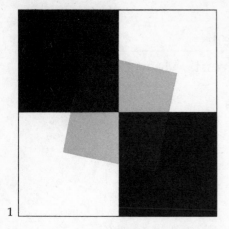

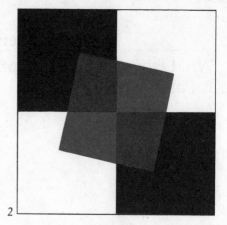

1

2

All other conditions being equal, the degree of similarity of the grays of the central region is the stimulus condition giving rise to a greater or lesser "degree of transparency." But what is the meaning of this expression? How do subjects support their description of greater or lesser transparency?

Descriptions obtained are of three types. When transparency is greater: (1) One sees what is beyond more clearly—the clarity of what is seen beyond is more striking, transparency is more "evident," "pronounced," "compelling." (2) The transparent layer is less visible. (3) What is beyond is less altered by the superposition of the transparent object.

As with any comparison, the difference in the degree of transparency may become so small as to reach threshold value. But whether one uses a series of filters or physically opaque models that give rise to perceptual transparency such as those described above, when differences in perceived transparency are not near the threshold, judgments of transparency are unanimous and are expressed with certainty. For example, no subject expresses doubt that Kodak wratten filter 96.20 is more transparent than wratten filter 96.80 when each of these filters is superimposed on a different part of the same checkerboard; nor is there any doubt about the greater transparency of the transparent layer perceived in Figure 1 as compared with the transparent layer perceived in Figure 2.

If other conditions also differ—for example, the color of the transparent layer (Figs. 3 and 4), or some feature of the surface perceived beyond the transparent layer, which may have a figure-ground organization (Fig. 5)—then the judgment may become more difficult and the threshold may rise; but there are still cases in which differences in perceived transparency are strong, and in these cases the consistency of the judgments remains.

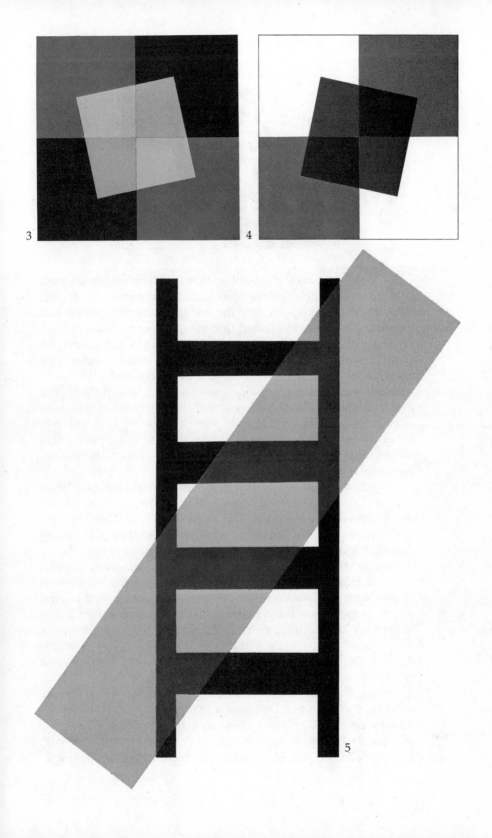

3

4

5

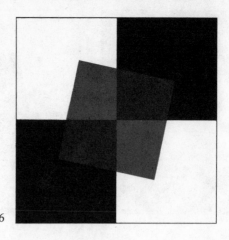

6

There is, however, a situation where subjects' judgments are contradictory, although the difference in transparency is evident. If the task is to compare the transparency of Figures 6 and 7 (and it has been established that subjects perceive a transparent layer or film covering the central region in both figures), we are faced with a disappointing result: some subjects assert that transparency is greater in Figure 6, some in Figure 7.

How are such contradictory results to be interpreted? The first hypothesis to be considered, that the difference in transparency is below (or near) threshold, can easily be rejected: subjects do not show uncertainty or difficulty in expressing their judgments, and judgments made by any given subject show a remarkable consistency.

Another hypothesis is that the same objective figure gives rise to different perceived figures, as often happens in experiments on visual perception. But in such cases sudden changes are experienced by subjects, who say that they are seeing "another thing" or another feature. This does not happen here.

Finally, the contradictory assertions of subjects may depend on an unclear definition of the task, so that subjects may be interpreting it in different ways. However, the task was the same when subjects were asked to compare the two transparent layers in Figure 1 and Figure 2, and in this case the subjects' judgments were consistent, showing that the task was clearly enough defined. It seems to have become insufficiently defined only when subjects were asked to compare Figures 6 and 7.

As has been noted above, when subjects are asked to specify what they mean when they assert that one film or filter is more transparent than another, they give three different reasons, which may be considered criteria for degree of transparency. If we compare the pair of transparent layers in Figures 1 and 2,

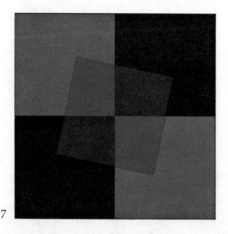

7

these criteria yield the same result: in Figure 1 one sees more clearly what is "beyond," the transparent layer is less visible, and what is seen beyond is less altered by the superposition of the transparent layer—that is, there is less difference between the protruding part of the ground or figure and the part of the ground or figure seen through the transparent layer. But when Figures 6 and 7 are compared, the three criteria give different results: they do not indicate the same figure as being the more transparent. In Figure 6 one sees more clearly what is beyond, while in Figure 7 the transparent layer is less visible and what is seen beyond is less altered by the interposition of the transparent layer. Thus it seems that a clearer criterion for the degree of transparency has to be found, one which avoids such inconsistent results.

If we follow this line of reasoning, however, and make the task more specific by telling subjects to use the criterion of the visibility of the transparent layer in judging degrees of transparency, complete agreement of subjects is still not reached. In fact there is an impressive perceptual quality present in Figure 6 but lacking in Figure 7—namely, the greater salience of the color-splitting phenomenon, which is more clean, more clear, and (in a sense) more beautiful. This aspect has to be disregarded if one wants to assert that there is more transparency in Figure 7.

The problem raised by the comparison of Figures 6 and 7 cannot, however, be considered settled by the preceding comments. There remains a problem of dimensionality in transparency. What must be clarified is whether transparency is a unidimensional or a bidimensional phenomenon—that is, whether transparency can vary independently in degree and salience or prägnanz, just as color can vary independently in hue, brightness, and saturation.

Fabio
Metelli

If the color of the transparent layer is held constant, the degree of transparency is measured by the index of chromatic scission α (Metelli, 1970, 1974 b):

$$\alpha = \frac{p-q}{a-b}$$

where p and q are the albedos of the splitting colors, while a and b are the albedos of the ground (black and white in Figs. 1, 2, and 6).

It is clear that if p and q become more similar and a and b remain unchanged, α decreases; this happens in Figure 2 (as compared with Figure 1) and, in fact, there is less transparency in Figure 2 than in Figure 1.

But α also varies if (p and q remaining unchanged) a and b become more similar, that is, if the $a-b$ difference decreases. In this case, since the denominator of the fraction decreases and the numerator remains unchanged, the value of α increases, and since the color of the transparent layer remains approximately equal, the prediction is that the degree of transparency increases. Figure 6 differs from Figure 7 only with respect to colors a and b, which are more different in Figure 6, being white and black, while they are light gray and dark gray in Figure 7. Therefore, according to the theory of perceptual splitting, transparency should be greater in Figure 7.

REFERENCES   Metelli, F. An algebraic development of the theory of perceptual transparency. *Ergonomics 13* (1970): 59–66.

Metelli, F. The perception of transparency. *Scientific American* (1974): 90–98. (a)

Metelli, F. Achromatic color conditions in the perception of transparency. In R.B. MacLeod & H.L. Pick, Jr. (Eds.), *Perception. Essays in honor of James J. Gibson*, 95–116. Ithaca, N.Y.: Cornell University Press, 1974. (b)

Metzger, W. *Gesetze des Sehens* (2d ed.). Frankfurt am Main: Waldemar Kramer Verlag, 1953.

Gaetano Kanizsa and Walter Gerbino

Convexity and Symmetry in Figure-Ground Organization

When the factors involved in perceptual organization are discussed, an important role is usually assigned to the tendency to maximal regularity, and, in particular, to that special case of regularity represented by the tendency to symmetry. In order to illustrate the influence of this factor, the patterns constructed by Bahnsen (1928), a student of Rubin, are often used. They are the designs he employed in studying the relation between symmetry and the division of the visual field into figure and ground. His demonstrations (Figs. 1 and 2) yield quite clear results: other things being equal, the regions of the visual field that have symmetric contours with respect to the vertical axis are seen as figures (rather than the regions lacking such symmetry).

Arnheim (1954) has pointed out that the factor of symmetry is not always sufficient to guarantee figure character to a given region. This will be the case when a further factor exerts its influence, such as the concavity of contours (Fig. 3), which has already been described by Rubin as supporting figure character. In Figure 3 both possible versions of figure and ground present symmetrical shapes, but these are convex in one of the versions, concave in the other. Although the configuration is quite unstable, Arnheim has asserted that the convex regions are more readily seen as figure.

It may be of interest, therefore, to study the influence of this important factor when it is in conflict with that of symmetry, especially since in Bahnsen's patterns the convexity of the contours has not, it seems to us, been sufficiently considered.

In the experiments described below we have tried to isolate and put into opposition these two factors in order to determine the role of each in figure-ground articulation.

As a preliminary step we have demonstrated once again the importance of convexity in the determination of figure and ground, 25

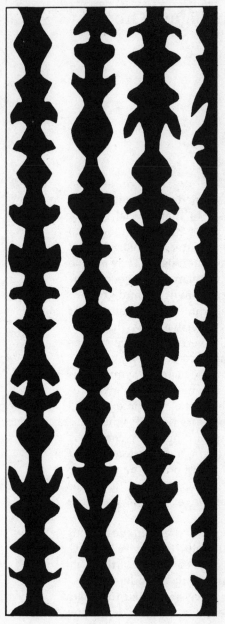

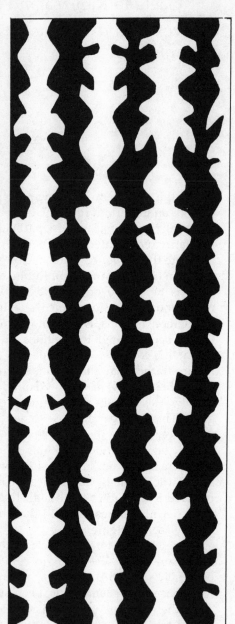

1

2

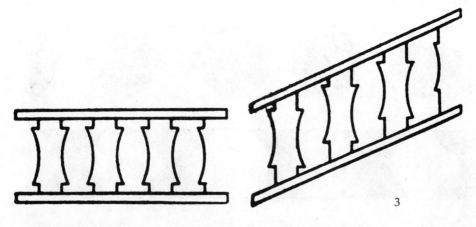

3

other things being equal with respect to symmetry. In Figure 4 both the white and the black regions are symmetric, but the white regions are primarily convex and the black ones primarily concave. The inverse is true in Figure 5. These patterns (15 x 16 cm) were mounted on gray cards and presented, one at a time, at a right angle to the line of sight of the subjects seated at a distance of 150 cm. We asked 40 subjects whether they saw "white figures on a black background or black figures on a white background." Half of the subjects were shown the patterns with the black margin to the left, and the other half saw the patterns with the white margin to the left.

The results are quite clear. In 74 out of 80 cases, subjects saw convex figures. Thus, other things being equal with respect to symmetry, regions with convex contours tend to prevail over those with concave contours in the determination of figures.

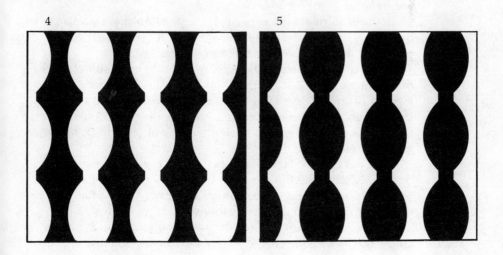

4   5

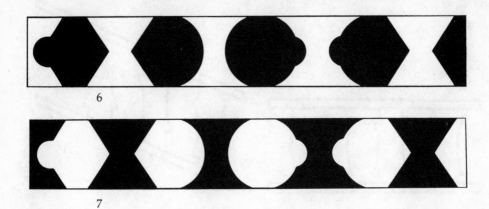

6

7

In order to put symmetry and convexity into direct opposition, we designed Figures 6 and 7 (2.5 x 15 cm), in which the regions with concave contours are symmetric with respect to both the vertical and horizontal axes, whereas the convex regions have a lower degree of symmetry. That is, the latter are symmetric only with respect to the horizontal axis which, as Mach (1911) observed, is a much less effective condition for producing the impression of symmetry than is symmetry with respect to the vertical axis.

In this case as well, the results are highly significant and demonstrate that convexity is much more important than symmetry in determining which region of the visual field is seen as figure. In 73 out of 80 cases, the convex areas were perceived as figures, whereas the symmetric areas did not have an independent existence, but rather became fused together so as to form a background.

In order to make the experimental situation more similar to Bahnsen's, we constructed Figures 8 and 10, with their corresponding "negative" versions, Figures 9 and 11.

This experiment was conducted with another 40 subjects, 20 of whom were shown Figures 8 and 9, while the other 20 saw Figures 10 and 11. In all four cases the patterns were 12 x 14 cm. In addition, half of the subjects were shown the patterns with the convex marginal area to the left. For the other half, this margin was to the right.

In 72 out of 80 observations, the convex regions were seen as figures. Neither the difference in brightness nor the placement to the left or the right of the convex marginal area had any detectable influence on the observations.

Completely analogous results were obtained in a further study in which Figures 8 and 9 were modified so that the area of

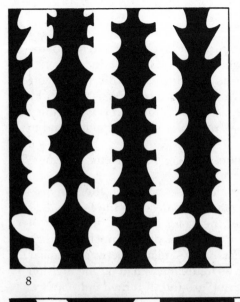

8

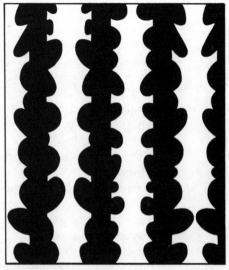

9

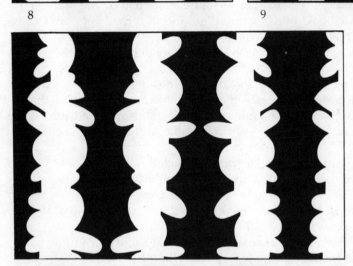

10

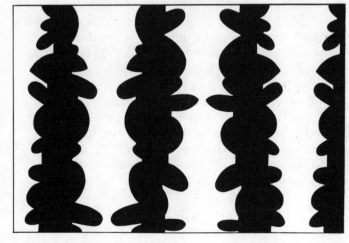

11

the symmetric regions was reduced by 20 percent and that of the corresponding regions of Figures 10 and 11 was reduced by 12.5 percent. This modification was introduced in order to promote the formation of the concave symmetric regions as figures by shifting the factor of relative size to their favor. It is well known that, other things being equal, relatively smaller regions tend to be seen as figures.

Even under these conditions, the convexity factor was more influential in 71 out of 80 observations.

At the end of each experimental session with the four patterns 8–11, the subjects were asked to describe the figures that they had seen, attributing to them, for example, some sort of meaning. This was done in order to determine how much influence past experience (that is, the similarity between familiar objects and the regions seen as figures) had had on the division of the visual field into figure and ground. It turned out that, except for a few cases, the convex figures were experienced as objects which possessed a strikingly three-dimensional character.

In considering this fact, we wondered whether our patterns were entirely appropriate for studying the influence of convexity on figure formation or whether, perhaps, the tendency of the convex regions to be seen as three-dimensional had added another factor which was also favorable to their being seen as figure.

To explore this problem, we constructed Figures 12 and 13 in which the regions with convex contours have a flatter appearance and less tendency to be seen in relief, even though it seems that there is a tendency, nevertheless, for such rounded and convex shapes to take on a more "bulky" appearance.

This experiment was conducted with the same procedure and with patterns measuring 8 x 15 cm. The results obtained from the 40 subjects are shown in Table 1.

As can be seen, the hypothesis that another factor, in addition to convexity, influenced the results reported above is somewhat supported by the results of this final experiment. In fact, the number of cases in which the convex regions are seen as figures is notably diminished (59 out of 80) and, in the case of Figure 12, this number is statistically much less significant.

In Figure 12 the dark color of the symmetric regions may have favored their being seen as figures. Indeed, according to some authors, brightness differences are an important aspect of figure-ground phenomena in the sense that, other things being equal, dark regions tend to be seen as figure and lighter regions

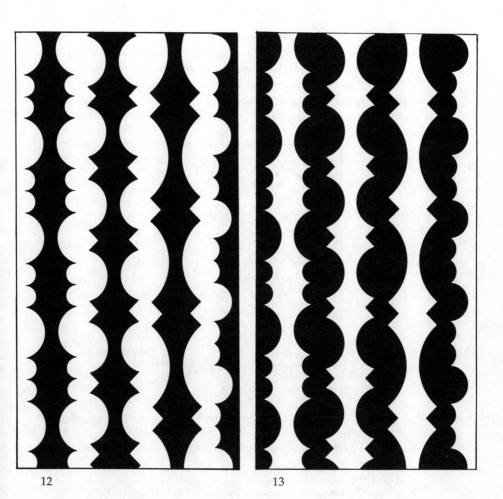

12   13

Table 1

Figure-Ground Organization: Convexity versus Symmetry

| Figure | Area Seen as Figure | | |
	Convex Asymmetric	Symmetric	Alternating
12	26*	8	6
13	33**	3	4
Total	59**	11	10

*$p < .05.$ **$p < .001.$

as ground. It might thus be of interest to conduct a systematic study of this factor by repeating the above-described experiments, but eliminating the differences in brightness. That is, one could replace our patterns, composed of juxtaposed black and white regions, by corresponding line drawings, as shown, for example, in Figure 14, which is the line drawing version of Figure 8.

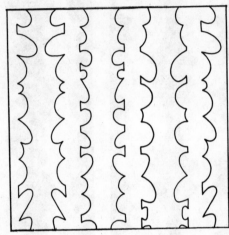

14

REFERENCES   Arnheim, R. *Art and visual perception*. Berkeley: University of California Press, 1954.

Bahnsen, P. Eine Untersuchung über Symmetrie und Asymmetrie bei visuellen Wahrnehmungen. *Zeitschrift für Psychologie 108* (1928): 129–154.

Kanizsa, G. The role of regularity in perceptual organization. In F. d'Arcais (Ed.), *Studies in perception*. Milan: Martello, 1974.

Mach, E. *Die Analyse der Empfindungen*. Jena, 1911.

Rubin, E. *Visuell wahrgenommene Figuren*. Copenhagen: Gyldendalske Boghandel, 1921.

John M. Kennedy

Attention, Brightness, and the Constructive Eye

My aim here is to suggest that attention can produce changes in the apparent brightness[1] of a surface. The mental process responsible may be, in part, a kind of "pictorial" attention. My subject matter is a strange one, called *subjective contours*, totally imaginary divisions mysteriously created by eye across uniform surfaces.

Subjective Contours

The term subjective contour[2] is used by Osgood (1953) for a kind of contour noticed by Schumann (1904) in Figure 1. At times an evanescent square can be seen, bordered by semicircles. The square's vertical sides are seen as complete by some people, and an occasional person can see the horizontal sides too, generally looking less definite than the vertical ones. Very few people see the square until they are instructed to look for it, and it generally takes a few minutes after the instructions are given before subjects can constitute the square. A particularly helpful device is to ask the subject to judge which region is brighter, the central square or the white arc bounded by the black semicircles; the white arc is often seen as the brighter, and the vertical sides of the square can be seen simultaneously. The sides of the evanescent square are "purely subjective" in the sense that there is no change in reflectance in the display corresponding to the perceived sides.

Schumann deserves credit for introducing subjective contours to perceptual psychology, but their full-scale investigation in recent years stems from the work of Kanizsa (1955). Figure 2 is one of Kanizsa's widely discussed figures involving strong contours (e.g., Coren, 1972; Varin, 1971; Gregory, 1972; Harris & Gregory, 1973). It is easier to see the bright subjective triangle in Figure 2 than the square in Figure 1.

33

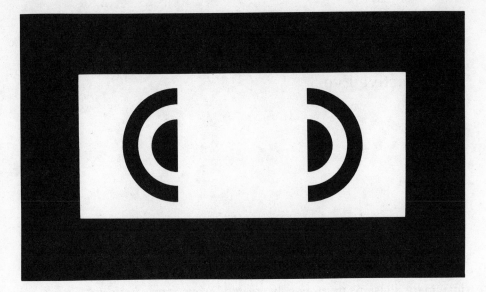

1
Schumann's
figure.

It is also possible to produce strong subjective contours with plain line figures, as in Figure 3 (from Kennedy, in press).

Are subjective contours a result of some simple spreading of excitation on the retina? Are peripheral mechanisms of attention, like eye movements, their cause? Or are they central, arising from mechanisms deeper in the sensorium?

It is difficult to account for subjective contours by purely retinal machinery. They can be produced by binocular displays, via disparity that creates *depth* (Julesz, 1964) and via two displays (Fig. 4) which summate to give subjective contours *without depth* (Kennedy & Chattaway, in preparation). Lateral inhibition, in the retinal, lower-order neurons, fails to predict the contour's shapes, and eye movement theories also fail because after-images show subjective contours.

3
Subjective
dividing
line.

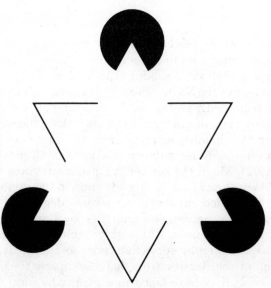

2   Kanizsa's triangle without corresponding gradients in the display.

4   Two part displays *(a,b)* that join binocularly to form the whole display *(c)*, which has a binocular subjective dividing line separating two coplanar regions.

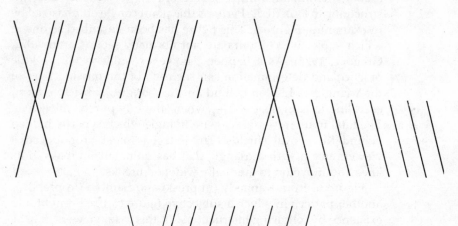

In fine, a central mechanism is involved, and in this vein the contours are often said to depend on the "closure" that governs the grouping of disconnected dots into a *line* of dots—the principle that allows the Vs in Figure 5 to be seen as a triangle. Alas (for this argument), seeing the Vs as a triangle usually occurs without any evidence of extra contours linking the outstretched arms of the Vs. Identifying an incomplete figure does not force a completion involving subjective contours (Kennedy, 1971; Coren, 1972). Might the key central mechanism be a kind of attention? What justifies invoking attention in this context?

First, as pointed out above, no lower-order retinal theory fits the phenomena. Second, no grouping laws are capable of explaining the phenomena. Although grouping laws explain some of the shapes taken by subjective contours (Kennedy, in press) and some of the depth effects that accompany these contours (Coren, 1972), they have failed to explain why form is seen directly and brightly in subjective contour displays, and incompletely in displays like Figure 5 seen as a triangle.

Third, instructions often play a central role in the genesis of these forms, a fact which calls convincingly for an attention theory. Schumann's inner square often appears only after instructions to look for it. Perhaps this point can be emphasized by re-examining Figure 5. This figure has been described as one in which subjective contours are not normally seen (Coren, 1972; Gregory, 1972). As it happens, however, subjects with a little practice and determination can see each of the missing lines of the triangle as hidden behind an oval, bright, subjective form, each line looking like —0—, where the 0 is purely subjective. The total figure resembles a wire triangle which is partly hidden behind three oval shields. This effect is most pronounced if viewers begin with a triangle that has quite small breaks in its lines and move on to gradually widened breaks.

Figure 6, from Kennedy (in press) and Sambin (in press), is another pattern in which a subjective figure can be brought into existence by following instructions. In this case, viewers may be asked to create a subjective circle whose perimeter touches the terminations of the lines, as though the lines were attachments to the central form.

A fourth reason for turning to attention explanations is the failure of contrast explanations. Neighboring regions often tend to enhance one another "by contrast," so that a white patch lying on a black field looks brighter than an identical white patch on a gray field. Schumann disputed contrast explanations of

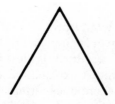

5   Vertices of a triangle or . . . ? The percept can change in accordance with instructions.

6   A subjective form can appear in the center of the lines.

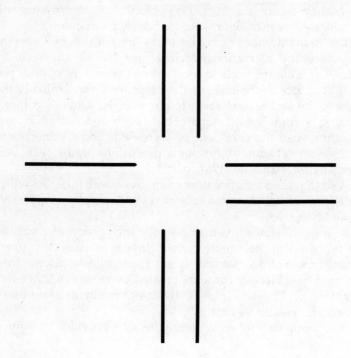

Figure 1, saying they would predict that the white arc almost surrounded by black would appear brightest, while he found that the interior square was the brightest region.

A sophisticated contrast explanation could argue that contrast is most marked where lines terminate or contours change direction. On this hypothesis, if several black line terminations (or contours changing direction) are grouped within a region (by the eye or by evident physical divisions), that region is uniformly enhanced,[3] showing subjective contours.

This hypothesis is also inadequate, for in Figure 7 lines have been added to Figure 5, enclosing the six line terminations, but the enclosed region is not uniformly brighter than the "exclosed" area.

A fifth reason to pursue an attention theory of subjective contours is their amenability to change, once formed.

The triangle figure (Fig. 5) is a good example. As Coren (1972) points out, with a little care one can achieve an impression of an inverted equilateral subjective triangle superimposed on the black line triangle. Thus Figure 5 can give rise to a subjective inverted triangle or to three "shields." The triangle and shields replace each other, just as one form replaces the other rather than superimposes itself on the other in reversible figures. Evidently the triangle figure is a reversible subjective contour figure, and the reversals of such figures are helped by instructions.

The radiating lines of Figure 6 also permit different shapes, encouraged by instructions. A circle form has already been described. It is also possible to see a strong square whose sides run at right angles to the lines of the objective figure. Initially the sides of the square may seem to curve at the square's corners, forming a rounded-off square but, with concentration, the straightness of the sides can be increased. Some subjects can also see an octagonal figure or a pincushion figure. (Cf. Berliner's figure, Arnheim, 1954, p.44.)

A sixth reason for appealing to attention is that factors which in themselves do not create subjective contours play a major role in modifying them.

Four equidistant dots may give the impression of a square, but the sides of the square do not appear as subjective lines. When, however, the same dots are appropriately placed, they can modify subjective contours created by means of other features (Fig. 8). The dots act as catalysts—they aid the effort to see a particular subjective form.

A seventh basis for an attention theory is provided by a study

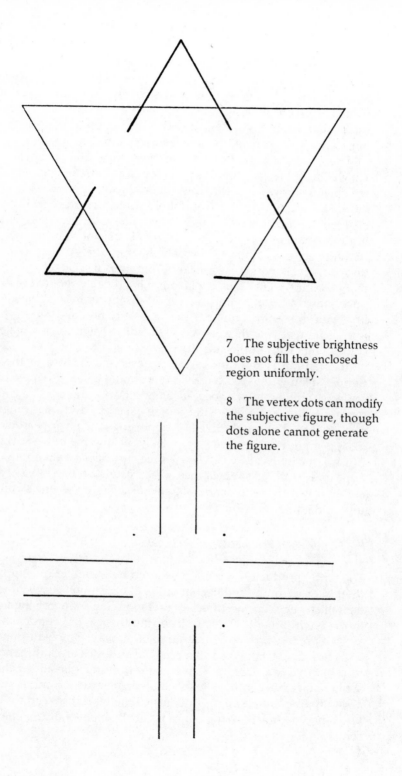

7   The subjective brightness
does not fill the enclosed
region uniformly.

8   The vertex dots can modify
the subjective figure, though
dots alone cannot generate
the figure.

of 10–11 year-olds who were asked to report on the disappearance and reappearance of subjective lines. Figure 3 was shown to the children. It was brought progressively closer until the line vanished; again, it was gradually moved away until the line re-established itself. (When the angular separation of the line terminations is very small, the line is unavoidable, compelling.)

There was a perceptual hysteresis effect: the distance at which the subjective line disappeared was *not* the distance at which it reappeared. A simple theory would predict that (1) once established, the line would hold up to a point close to the observer, and (2) once lost, the line would not re-establish itself until the display was taken to a favorable distance farther away from the observer. In fact, precisely the opposite was found: the disappearance point was *farther* from the observer than the reappearance point.[4] The explanation is probably the following: once subjects are *set* to find and report disappearance, subjective lines vanish readily, and once they are *set* to find and report the line again, reappearance also occurs readily. Attention is a major controlling factor in the stability of the line.

If attention is relevant to the genesis and demise of these figures, even with children, then one should be able to increase *or* decrease the rate of appearance and disappearance. The children from the hysteresis study were asked to do three things: one, to gaze at the subjective line, reporting when it appeared or disappeared; two, to *speed up*—quickly making the line go away if it was present and vice versa; three, to *slow down* the rate of appearance and disappearance. The results showed that the children were able to accelerate and decelerate the line's comings and goings at will.

Productive Attention and Ways of Looking

The term "productive attention" is used here to refer to a hypothetical process, the architect of optional perceptual effects, ones for which there are no directly corresponding inhomogeneities in the environment. Delving deep into theory, let us ask what kind of process it is, as compared to other ways of looking.

Schumann established that analytic attitudes are antithetical to bjective contours (cf. Kanizsa, 1974). It must be added that some subjective contours resist analytic destruction more successfully than others, e.g., in Figure 9 the black bars cannot be weakened as much as the contours at the elbows of the chevrons.

Schumann's observation is a strange one. It implies that when we are asked to be analytic, to determine what is truly there, we are often able to pick out the veridical lines and marks, distinguishing them from the subjective ones and weakening the subjective ones as a result. Even children have volunteered observations on this point: for example Fiona (age 9), who said quite plainly, "I see a line that isn't there." Describing what they see in Figure 3, subjects young and old quite spontaneously, without any pertinent prodding, often remark that some lines are *there* and some are *imaginary*.[5] In the absence of any leading questions beyond "What do you see here?" the displays allow subjects, even young subjects, to make epistemological distinctions between appearance and reality, and the subjective lines are classified as "appearance"— subjectively subjective, as it were. In sum, the genesis of these forms involves a nonanalytic kind of attention, generating imaginary things often known to be precisely that, imaginary.

Besides analytic attention, Gibson and the Gestalt psychologists distinguish ways of looking that are direct and immediate—"looking näively without bias at the facts of im-

9 Contours at the elbows of the white chevrons are more labile than the subjective black bars.

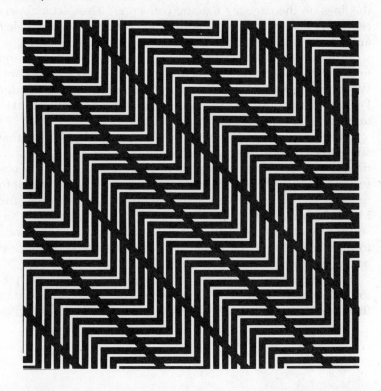

mediate experience" (Koffka, 1935, p. 73; cf. Kolers, 1972, p. 160)—a kind of looking akin to Gibson's "visual world" impressions. Within the visual world attention has a role, for one can look in different directions, sampling different parts of the environment.

Are subjective contours a result of a visual world way of looking? It seems not. We may look at Figure 5, for example, then off to the side, then back again, several times— attending to it, then directing our attention elsewhere for a moment. This sampling kind of attention does not favor the emergence of subjective contours. Instructions to create the figure *without* altering the *direction* of attention are much more useful.

In sum, neither the visual world concept, with its sampling attention, nor analytic ways of looking can explain the effects of productive attention.

Productive Attention and Pictorial Perception

Continuing with theory, let us take an unusual step and compare subjective contours with the special perception used for simple line sketches.

Seeing a hasty sketch, we say, "I see a face, but literally it's only a few lines," or "I see parallel tracks receding, but actually the lines on the page are flat and converge." This pictorial perception is *dual* or *bicameral*, a double percept of an outlined *object* and a few *lines* with a different shape and location.

It is commonplace that the sides (lengths) of contours and lines may be "surrogates" (Hochberg, 1962) for depth and slant. What can the *ends* of lines and *changes in direction* of contours do? Perhaps they can support *pictorial* impressions of *brightness* akin to the *pictorial depth* of the sides of lines.

At heart, a pictorial hypothesis is suggested by the fact that subjective contours need not be illusory. By definition, geometric illusions give erroneous percepts, impressions that the observer finds convincing. We need operations of measurement to tell us that we are misled about length in, for example, the Müller-Lyer illusion. By contrast, in simple line pictures the observer can tell that the pictured depth is not veridical; there is no trompe l'oeil. Similarly, subjective contours can be seen, even by children, not to be truly present.

Simple patterns like Rubin's figure-ground displays are pictorial (Kennedy, 1974), and the depth relationships perceived in them are optional, not inevitable (Kennedy, 1973). Similarly, in simple patterns subjective contours are often optional, requiring instructions to bring them forward.

Pictorial form and depth are malleable; in particular, they are often reversible (multistable, in Attneave's [1971] phrase). So too, subjective contours are malleable in form, *and reversible* at times. Schumann's figure can be seen in the way Schumann reported, with the central square as the brightest region. Or the brightness step from the square to the almost enclosed white

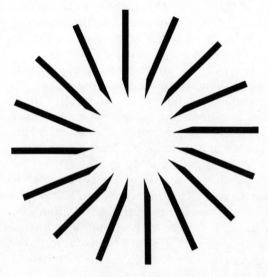

10   The central subjective figure readily reverses from light to dark, particularly in peripheral vision.

arcs can be reversed, so that the arcs seem to be the brightest region. (Personally, I am unable to achieve this figure's reversal, but 7 of 8 adult subjects I tested assured me that they could.) Shipley (1965) found "anomalous" brightness reversals in binocular displays that produced subjective contour squares. Figure 10 is reversible; usually it is seen, on first exposure, as luminous in the center, with an ill-defined margin. (On occasion it has been seen on first exposure as dark in the center—notably by a prominent biologist accustomed to microscopic viewing of dark circular spores with appendages.) To make Figure 10 reverse in brightness, it is often helpful to look to the side of the figure, at the region outside the radiating lines, while attending to the center; a dark, textured disc or ball will seem to alternate with the luminous appearance.

John M. Kennedy

To predict which subjective contour figures will reverse in brightness, and when, is an uncertain business. But most subjects can reverse some figures, and binocularly defined contours are probably quite easy to reverse since there are no strong monocular effects to oppose potential reversals. Also, monocular figures like that in Figure 3, where monocular effects are equipoised on either side of the subjective line, can probably be quite readily reversed in brightness once one has seen one adjoining region as darker than the other. The actual subjective line in Figure 3 has an indefinite brightness, sometimes dark, sometimes light, and often a mixture along the length of the figure, dark for a stretch and light for a stretch.

In sum, just as adjoining regions can appear with reversible pictorial depth relations, so too adjoining regions may have reversible brightness relations. Pictorial depth can reverse even when one of the alternating percepts is more regular, recognizable, and probable than the other (Rubin, 1915; Howard, 1961; Kennedy, 1974), and pictorial brightness can also reverse even when very powerful, as Figure 10 indicates.

Pictorial depth can appear without the aid of recognizable form or specific depth cues in the display. Rubin's displays were "nonsense forms," yet depth steps (stratification) could be seen. Similarly, subjective contours need not have a regular form or define a familiar object. It would be wrong to take their occasional irregular shape or unrecognizable pattern as a reason for rejecting a pictorial hypothesis.

In all, there are many affinities between pictorial depth and subjective contour brightness. Just as our eye uses flat outline sketches to see the surface arrangements we call "depth" and "slant" (Kennedy, 1974), so too our eye uses line and contour sketches to see the features of surfaces that we call "change of brightness"; and detailed parallels to change of brightness due to cracks, pigment, opaque surfaces, and transparent surfaces (Varin, 1971; Kanizsa, 1974; Kennedy, in press) can be drawn. To unite in one demonstration both pictorial depth and pictorial brightness, consider that a quite flat picture can show a surface bulging out or caving in. Will subjective contours conform to pictorial space *in the picture* or to the physical flatness of the perceived surface *of the picture*?

If the pictorial interpretation of the modus operandi of subjective contours is correct, the subjective region should conform to the pictured space. That is, between the subjective contours an entire surface should be generated, bright as usual, but

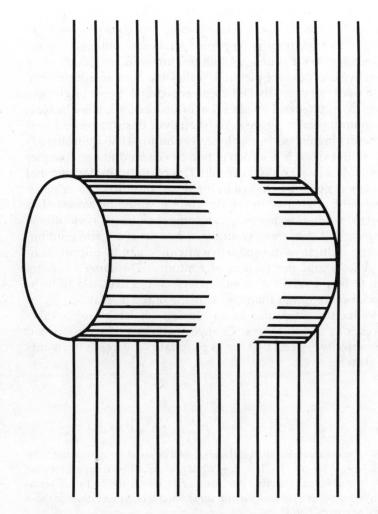

11   The subjective central stripe lies in three-dimensional pictorial space, not the flat space of the physical display.

three-dimensional, although the eye can tell that the depth is only pictorial. Figure 11 seems to provide the predicted result. A pictured cylinder is evident, partly defined by a line gradient, and where the lines end a subjective shape appears in the form of the continuation of the cylinder. The subjective surface belongs in the pictorial space, *not* as background conforming to the perceived flatness of the display's surface. The cylindrical subjective band is opaque, bowed outwards, clearly a depicted surface in the depicted space.

John M.
Kennedy

Thus the mechanism for many subjective contours seems to be a kind of pictorial perception, paralleling outlined figure-ground depth. Of course, not all brightness discriminations or subjective contours are pictorial, just as the existence of pictorial depth does not show that all depth is pictorial. Some brightness effects do not depend on attention or instructions; some subjective contours, as in Figure 9, resist analytic destruction and cannot be distinguished from physical contours. The claim here is that, at times, brightness perception can be modified so that pictorial (subjective) contours result. The opportunity for pictorial contours is given by change in the reflectance of a line or patch of pigment or change in the direction of a line or border. The changes, when *close together*, can compel us to see nonoptional (nonpictorial) subjective contours; when *far apart*, the guiding, molding influences of productive attention can be important in the genesis and destruction of contours. The latter contours seem to be pictorial, to be subjectively subjective, and to lie in pictorial space rather than on the plane of the display.

Productive attention, in conclusion, develops remarkable impressions of brightness. Changes in lines and contours can give subjective effects that are as pictorial as the depth in an outline sketch.

NOTES   1. The colloquial term "brightness" will be used here for what technically might be called reflectance, whiteness, or albedo, in part for ease of style and in part because the manner in which the technical terms apply to subjective contours is still undecided. For a discussion of these terms, see Beck (1974).

2. Kanizsa (1974) counsels avoiding this term in favor of "contours without gradients." However, as will be seen, the term "subjective" nicely indicates the fact that naïve subjects often judge these contours, lines, and gradations to be purely subjective.

3. To account for the uniform appearance of Kanizsa's triangle (Fig. 2), which is equally bright near to and far from the physically present black regions, it is necessary to assume that inducing contrast effects act uniformly throughout any enclosed perceptual region, even though the inducing line terminations, etc. are concentrated at the periphery of the enclosed region.

4. The disappearance point was 35.8 inches (mean for 12 subjects), and the corresponding reappearance point was 27.8 inches (same subjects) with $p < 01$. The number of children able to *speed up* disappear-

ance and reappearance was 10 out of 12, while 7 were able to *slow down* the rate, and 2 were faster when asked to slow down.

5. That is, the 10–11 year-olds were not asked any question that included terms like "appearance," "reality," "really there," "looks like," or "seems like." They were simply asked to say what they saw, and they spontaneously introduced the distinction between reality and appearance, what was real and what was imaginary.

It is very unusual in psychology to take the subject's phenomenological epistemology into consideration. The exceptional attempts to do so, by Gibson, Bozzi, and some Piagetians, have been treated gingerly at best. When it is as consistently and strongly stated as here by naïve subjects, children, without leading questions, there is no way to avoid it—and the sooner we take it seriously the better!

REFERENCES

Arnheim, R. *Art and visual perception.* Berkeley: University of California Press, 1954.

Attneave, F. Multistability in perception. *Scientific American 135* (1971): 62–71.

Beck, J. Dimensions of an achromatic surface color. In R.B. MacLeod & H. Pick (Eds.), *Perception: Essays in honor of James J. Gibson.* Ithaca: Cornell University Press, 1974.

Coren, S. Subjective contours and apparent depth. *Psychological Review 79* (1972): 359–367.

Gregory, R.L. Cognitive contours. *Nature 238* (1972): 51–52.

Harris, J.P., & Gregory, R.L. Fusion and rivalry of illusory contours. *Perception 2* (1973): 235–247.

Hochberg, J.E. The psychophysics of pictorial perception. *Audiovisual Communication Review 10* (1962): 22–54.

Howard, I.P. An investigation of a satiation process in the reversible perspective of revolving skeletal shapes. *Quarterly Journal of Experimental Psychology 13* (1961): 19–33.

Julesz, B. *The cyclopean eye.* New York: Random House, 1964.

Kanizsa, G. Marzini quasi-percettivi in campi con stimolazione omogenea. *Rivista di Psicologia 49* (1955): 7–30.

Kanizsa, G. Contours without gradients or cognitive contours? *Italian Journal of Psychology 1* (1974): 93–113.

Kennedy, J.M. Incomplete pictures and detection of features. *Journal of Structural Learning 1* (1971): 71–73.

Kennedy, J.M. Misunderstandings of figure and ground. *Scandinavian Journal of Psychology 14* (1973): 207–209.

Kennedy, J.M. *A psychology of picture perception: Images and information.* San Francisco: Jossey-Bass, 1974.

John M.
Kennedy

Kennedy, J.M. Depth at an edge, coplanarity, slant depth of subjective contours, *Italian Journal of Psychology*, in press.

Kennedy, J.M., & Chattaway, L.D.Subjective contours, binocular and movement phenomena. In preparation.

Koffka, K. *Principles of Gestalt psychology*. New York: Harcourt, Brace, 1935.

Kolers, P. *Aspects of motion perception*. New York: Pergamon Press, 1972.

Osgood, C.E. *Method and theory in experimental psychology*. New York: Oxford University Press, 1953.

Rubin, E. *Synsoplevede figurer*. Copenhagen: Glydendels, 1915.

Sambin, M. Angular margins without gradient. *Italian Journal of Psychology*, in press.

Schumann, F. Einige Beobachtungen über die Zusammenfassung von Gesichtseindrücken zu Einheiten. *Psychologische Studien 1* (1904): 1–32.

Shipley, T. Visual contours in homogeneous space. *Science 150* (1965): 348–350.

Varin, D. Fenomeni de contrasto e diffusione cromatica nell' organizzazione spaziale del campo percettivo. *Rivista di Psicologia 65* (1971): 101–128.

Dorothea Jameson and Leo M. Hurvich

From Contrast to Assimilation:
In Art and in the Eye

A central problem for psychologists has always been the issue of perceptual constancies. How do we recognize objects despite changes in perspective, changes in distance, changes in lighting, and so on? How do we recognize the surface characteristics of objects, and thus the objects themselves, despite relatively large changes in level of illumination and in the spectral quality of the lighting? A favorite example is the lump of coal that looks black and the white shirt that looks white when they are seen either outdoors on a bright sunny day or indoors under a 25-watt lamp, even though the amount of light reflected to the eye from the lump of coal outdoors is many times greater than the light reflected from the white shirt indoors under the 25-watt lamp. And the white shirt is recognized as white when it is outdoors and reflects the illumination from the sky into the eye, even though the skylight is heavily weighted in energy from the short wave region of the visible spectrum, the wave lengths that we think of as blue. It is still identified as white indoors under the incandescent lamp even though the light then has very little energy in the short wave spectral region and is heavily weighted in long wave energy that we usually think of as orange or reddish in hue.

This kind of constancy of brightness and color hue suggests that we directly perceive reflectance characteristics of surfaces rather than responding to the qualities of light in different parts of the light image that is in the eye. A rather common restatement, if not explanation, of this principle is that we respond to ratios of lights rather than to their amounts (Wallach, 1948). We know, of course, that the pupil of the eye enlarges when the illumination level is weak and contracts when it is strong, and

This article appeared in *Leonardo* 8 (Spring 1975): 125–131. Copyright © by Pergamon Press Ltd., Oxford. Reprinted by permission.

49

this compensatory change in the aperture of the eye does help to reduce the range of light levels to which the sensitive retina of the eye is exposed. Changes in pupil size alone, however, are by no means large enough to compensate for any but a small fraction of the range of illumination levels that control the amount of light imaged on the retina. Much more important is the mechanism that allows the retina to adjust its sensitivity to adapt to the prevailing light levels. When the prevailing level of illumination is strong, the retina becomes manyfold less light sensitive than it is when the prevailing illumination level is weak. Moreover, the retina not only adjusts its overall light sensitivity, it also adjusts the balance of sensitivities in the *different* retinal mechanisms that respond more or less selectively to light from different wave length regions of the visible energy spectrum. This relative sensitivity adjustment changes the color balance of the retina, again in such a way as to compensate for changes in the spectral weighting of the prevailing quality of illumination. But changes in pupil size and changes in sensitivities are such that they preserve *ratios* of light or responses to light within the image surface.

In short, we know that there are dynamic changes in both the level and the balance of sensitivities in the eye that *could*, if they were perfectly adjusted, perfectly compensate for any changes in quantity and spectral quality of illumination, and such perfectly compensatory dynamic sensitivity adjustments would lead us to expect complete constancy of surface brightness and color. Illumination information would simply be lost.

But of course this is not true. Our perceptual world may indeed be *recognizable* under a variety of illuminations, but the perceived constancy mechanism is not so perfect that it prevents us from knowing when we want to put on sunglasses, or when we want to change that 25-watt bulb for a 100-watt one. Does this mean simply that the sensitivity changes we have been discussing are only partly, rather than completely, compensatory? If this were the whole explanation, then an artist should be able to paint the same scene twice, and in the second, by slightly increasing the lightness throughout, to create an impression of much stronger illumination. But again, this is not the case.

Perhaps no group of artists knew the fascination of the non-constancy of our visual world better than the Impressionists, and Claude Monet's masterly renderings of the Rouen Cathedral, at different times of day and in different kinds of weather, are stunning examples of variation rather than constancy. Figure

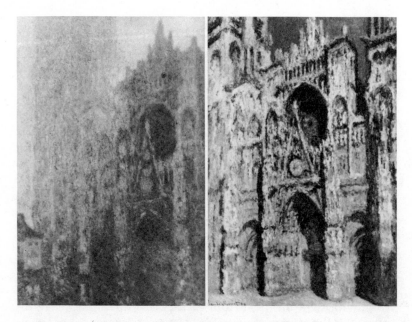

1   Claude Monet, *Early Morning* and *Afternoon, Full Sun*.

1 reproduces two of the Cathedral series in black and white photographs, and even in this impoverished form, the reader should have no great difficulty in deciding which of the two canvases represents the cathedral in dim, early-morning light and which in afternoon, full sun. The two versions, as reproduced here, differ little, if at all, in overall average reflectance. They do differ in two other important respects: the light areas are lighter and the dark areas darker in *Afternoon* than in *Early Morning*, and the contours where the lighter and darker areas meet appear sharper in *Afternoon* than in *Early Morning*. (For the moment we can ignore other differences, such as form and location of shadows, which indisputably provide clues from which we can deduce the most probable location of the sun in the sky, not to mention the subtleties of hue coloration that characterize the paintings and that are lost in the photographs.) If, in fact, we always perceive surface reflectance correctly, then changes in relative amounts of light in different parts of the scene would seem naturally to be somehow attributable to changes in illumination rather than to changes in surface properties. But do we always perceive surface reflectance correctly? What of Figure 2, which shows two identical gray surfaces embedded in two different backgrounds? The figure is adapted from a color illustration in Josef Albers' *Interaction of Color*, and the fundamental

principle that it illustrates is almost a universal starting point for anyone working with color, whether in art, design, perceptual psychology, or even visual physiology. Although there was a time in the history of perceptual psychology (Beck, 1972) when there might have been a pitting of points of view about the basis for simple contrast phenomena of the sort illustrated in Figure 2, we now know enough about the eye and the physiological properties of the visual system to be able to describe with some assurance how the visual neural network is organized so as to bring about such perceived contrast effects as a natural outcome of its dynamic functional organization.

Figure 3 is a diagrammatic representation of the human or primate retina taken from the work of Polyak (1941); it illustrates quite well the kinds of cells the microscopist can see in a cross section of the human retina. There are rods and cones, the receptors which contain the visual pigments that absorb the light locally incident on them from each part of the light image focused on the retina, a layer of bipolar cells, the retinal ganglion cells whose electrical spike discharges are transmitted up the fibers of the optic nerve to the brain centers, and also, in between these cells, the so-called horizontal cells between the receptors and bipolar layers. The diagram of Figure 4 is taken from the more recent work of Dowling and Boycott (1966), and it shows more clearly how the different retinal elements are interconnected. The rod and cone receptor cells make synaptic connections with the bipolars, and usually not simply in a one-to-one fashion. But note that the horizontal cell processes extend over relatively wide distances of the receptor cell mosaic, making multiple interconnections throughout, and there seems to be a similar broad system of multiple interconnections by way of the amacrine cells farther on in the pathway between bipolar and ganglion cells. With this picture in mind, it should hardly surprise us that light falling on one part of the retina should have some effect on what is seen in another part. Nor is it surprising to learn that if, in an animal preparation, a recording electrode is inserted in a single one of these ganglion cells, a small probe light moved across the retina can influence the electrical activity recorded from this ganglion cell when the position of the probe light is shifted from one receptor location to another. The total extent on the retina within which such a probe light can influence the electrical response activity of any particular single ganglion cell is called the "receptive field" of that ganglion cell. However, it is not simply the fact of that inter-

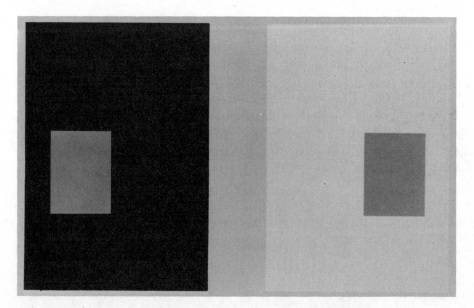

2   Two identical gray surfaces appear to differ in lightness because of contrast with their different surrounds.

3   Diagram of retina showing varieties of cells and interconnections among cells that are all involved in the eye's physiological response to a light image. Numbers differentiate anatomical layers and zones, letters refer to cell types. After Polyak (1941).

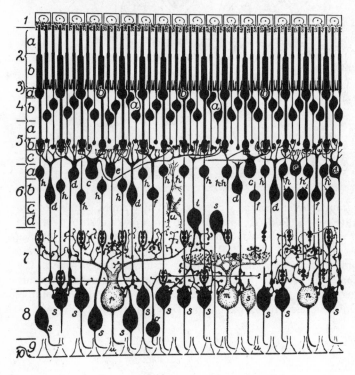

relatedness, but the nature of the interaction within the receptive field that is of most interest, because the nature of the interaction turns out to be precisely the kind needed to account for the contrast effects we perceive, and, in fact, the kind that some visual theorists assumed to exist long before the electrical activities of such single cells were ever measured (Ratliff, 1965).

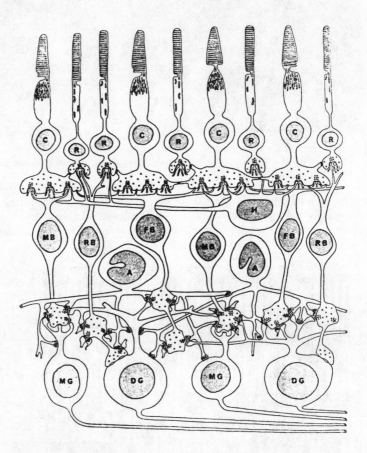

4 Diagram showing complex organization of synaptic connections in vertebrate retina. Rod (R) and cone (C) receptors absorb light and influence activity of bipolar cells (MB, RB, FB), and these influence activity of ganglion cells (MG, DG), whose spike discharges are transmitted along optic nerve fibers to visual centers in brain. The simultaneously activated horizontal (H) and amacrine (A) cells modify activities in different receptor-optic nerve pathways through multiple lateral interconnections. Diagram from Dowling and Boycott (1966).

This kind of spatial response is shown in Figure 5, which illustrates what v. Békésy (1968) has called a "neural unit." What is diagrammed is the response of a single cell when a probe light is moved across a region of the retina. Such a cell is spontaneously active in the dark when there is no light image on the retina. If a small light is turned on, the cell will increase its firing

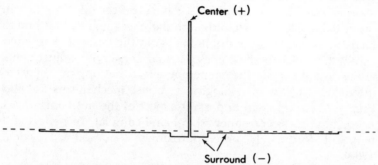

Center (+)

Surround (−)

5 Diagrammatic representation of response pattern of single cell to light imaged in different regions of retina. Surround responses (−) are opposite to center responses (+).

rate (indicated by the + sign in the diagram) when the light is imaged on that part of the retina which happens to be located at the center of the cell's retinal receptive field. When the light is moved a little way on the retina out of the central excitatory location, the electrical spiking in the cell is diminished to a firing rate less than the spontaneous activity rate (indicated by the − sign in the diagram), and if the light is strong enough, it will inhibit the spiking completely, so that the cell becomes silent. When the light is now turned off, the cell will respond with a burst of afterdischarge. Another cell may show the obverse behavior— namely, spiking to stimulation of the outer regions of its retinal receptive field and suppression of spiking, followed by afterdischarge, when the light goes off in the center. In either case, what we see is an antagonistic system of influences on the cell in a cell-surround spatial organization. We can now think of the retinal tissue as made up of systems of organized neural units, with the organizing principle one of spatial antagonism that is ideally suited to accentuate differences between adjacent parts of the retinal image in converting this image to a visual perception—a physiological contrast mechanism.

Jameson & Hurvich

We know from perception experiments with intact humans that the incremental opponent activities that serve as contrast sharpening mechanisms are stronger when the light stimulates the antagonistically interacting parts of the retina more strongly, and thus the contrast sharpening effect is greater when the overall level of illumination is increased (Jameson & Hurvich, 1961; Stevens, 1961). This is what we associate with the increased level of illumination: blacker blacks, whiter whites, sharper boundaries. Monet must have perceived the effect in order to be able to use it, although there was no need for him to have any knowledge or intuitions about the basis of sharpened contrast in visual physiology. Visual sensitivity adjustments alone do not explain the crispening effect, but opponent spatial interactions in the physiological response mechanisms do, and this, we believe, is an important aspect of the mechanism that keeps brightness constancy from being complete or perfect and makes it, fortunately, only approximate (Jameson & Hurvich, 1964).

The retinal principle of antagonistic organization is equally apparent, moreover, in the way the system is organized to give us color vision (Hurvich & Jameson, 1957; DeValois, 1973). To review that system briefly, light is absorbed selectively from different parts of the visible energy spectrum by three kinds of cone receptors containing different photopigments, one which absorbs light maximally in the short wave lengths, another that absorbs light maximally from the mid-spectrum, and a third with maximal absorption in the longer wave lengths. The different receptor activities initiated by light absorption in the three different photopigments eventually serve to activate three different kinds of cell systems: in one, the three kinds of inputs have the same effect on the cell; these summate, the information about different regions of the spectrum is lost, and such a cell probably simply codes brightness, or blackness, whiteness, and the gray scale in between. Its only antagonistic principle is the antagonistic center-surround spatial organization. In another, qualitatively different cell system, the inputs that derive from the different kinds of cones maintain their specificity, in the sense that one kind of input stimulates the cell to fire more rapidly, whereas another suppresses its firing rate. These have been called "spectrally opponent" cells. If the two inputs are perfectly matched in their antagonistic effects on the cell, they will cancel each other, and no "color coded" response will occur. If the antagonistic effects do not perfectly cancel each other, the particular hue presumably coded in the message sent to the brain will depend on whether the firing rate has increased or decreased from the spontaneous level when the eye was in darkness. All the evidence we have from analyzing our color perceptions, when combined with electrical records obtained from single visual nerve cells in various animals, suggests that there are two kinds of such hue coding systems, one for red versus green, and another for yellow versus blue (Hurvich & Jameson, 1957; DeValois, 1973).

The organization of the color vision mechanisms into three basic physiological systems, one reporting on white or black, one reporting yellow or blue, and a third reporting green or red, is an instance of what is called "parallel processing" in the nervous system. We shall return to this notion of parallel processing.

If we now remember that not only the white versus black, but also the qualitatively opponent yellow versus blue and red versus green hue systems are also organized into spatially opponent, center-surround neural units, we come to the physiological basis for spatial hue contrast (Jameson & Hurvich, 1964). Thus, for the same reason that a white background causes an enclosed gray surface to look blackish, a red background causes it to look greenish, and a blue background causes it to look yellowish.

Monet used the principle of hue contrast with particular effectiveness in his *Haystack* series; here he especially took advantage of the hue contrast phenomenon known as the colored shadow effect. We "know" it is a bright summer day when we see in one of these paintings the yellow of the sunlight on the left of the haystack and the strong blue of the shadow on the right. The colored shadow has a double basis. There is less yellow sunlight in the shadow area, but there is also a strong blue contrast component in the less strongly illuminated shadow area that comes about physiologically because of the opponent spatial organization of the yellow versus blue hue-coded neural units of the visual system. Monet has probably exaggerated the effect, but in doing so he has caught one of the essences of what we see in full sunlight.

Josef Albers (1963) has, of course, made full use of these contrast effects that he knows so well in his many series of paintings in *Homage to the Square*. In one example, which he calls *Homage to the Square "Assured,"* he achieves maximal blackness in the central element by surrounding black with white; in another, *Homage to the Square–Insert*, the same white surrounds a yellow center square, and, in this instance, by suppressing whiteness in the center, he increases the saturation or hue strength of the central yellow. In another series, he creates a perceptible step where the pigment has none. A broad, uniformly painted area that abuts a lighter area on one side and a darker one on the other will, if observed carefully, show a subtle contrast gradient. It looks darker where it abuts the lighter boundary and lighter where the boundary relations are reversed, with a scarcely noticed shading in between. By superimposing a sharp white contour line midway across the gradient, a step is created, with two relatively uniform areas appearing respectively as lighter and darker on either side of the contour.

Figure 6 reproduces a composition by Victor Vasarely (1970) which incorporates a subtle difference in contrast between tangent and abutting elements at the corners as opposed to the intermediate elements along any one uniformly pigmented line. The result is an intersecting pair of softly outlined, but luminously glowing, axes that are generated as pure physiological contrast light.

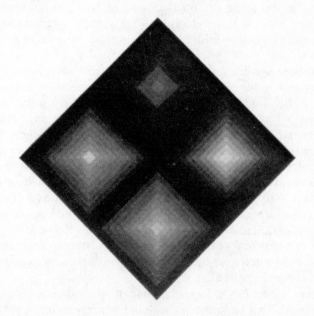

6   Vasarely composition (1970) in which "glowing" axes are generated by physiological contrast mechanisms of visual system. The original painting is executed in four different colors.

Contrast effects are effects of spatial interactions, and spatial interactions imply a dependence on spatial dimensions. If these dimensions become sufficiently small, as in the separately painted and differently colored dots of a pointillist painting, then contrast gives way to spatial mixture. If we stand at a sufficient distance from a painting such as Seurat's *Grande Jatte*, the size of the individual pigment dots is so small, and the grain of adjacent image elements on the retina is so fine, that they are not resolved as separate elements, but rather blend as in a superimposed light mixture. This was, of course, the theory on which the technique was based—namely, that light could be captured more effectively by using the principle of optical mixture to yield an additive mixture of lights reflected from the pigment elements rather than to rely on the standard procedure of subtractive pigment mixture by blending the colors on a palette. The principle here is trivial from the point of view of visual physiology and mechanisms of visual perception. The eye, like any optical system, has limited resolving power, and even people lucky enough to have perfectly normal uncorrected vision are unable to read the bottom line on an acuity chart if they stand too far away from it. At some distance, the tiny blurred images of the letters simply blend into one another or shade into the background, just as in a pointillist painting viewed at a comparable distance. At viewing distances shorter than that limit, however, there are letter sizes and image grains such that one can see that there are letters there, or where the pigment texture is obvious, but at which neither letters nor pigment dots are individually identifiable. The image dimensions in this region become of interest because they set the lower boundary of dimensions in which we perceive assimilation rather than contrast effects.

Assimilation effects are referred to as "optical mixture" by Albers (1963), but we prefer to reserve the term "optical mixture" for situations in which we do not have spatial resolution and mixture at the same time, because it is the paradox of simultaneous resolution and mixture that makes the phenomenon of special interest. The effect is sometimes also called "reversed contrast," an accurate descriptive term; it is often referred to by students of perception as the "Bezold Spreading Effect" (Evans, 1944), after Bezold (1876), who both described and illustrated it in his book on *Theory of Color*. Bezold's illustrations include a rather complex arabesque tracery superimposed on a continuous colored strip as background. If the pattern is done in black, the background too looks dark, and if the pattern is white, the background is also lightened. The background and pattern colors seem to shift toward each other, as if mixing, despite the fact that the contours remain quite distinct and well above the theshold of spatial resolution.

A contemporary painter whose work often combines both optical mixture and assimilation effects to generate new hues from a limited palette is Richard Anuszkiewicz, who studied with Albers. One example, entitled *Elemental Fire*, is a geometric composition based on three pigments: orange, white, and yellow. The outer limits of the geometric form are made up of solid orange rectangles and squares, diagonally oriented and touching at the corner points to form a complete enclosure. Within the enclosure, the same orange is alternated with white in equally spaced narrow stripes, and in the very center is a diamond made up of stripes of the same orange alternated with yellow ones. Where the repetitive pattern of stripes occurs, the orange seems to blend with the white or with the yellow so as to deny completely its "objective" identity with the solid orange of the outer parts of the pattern. Viewed from afar, the separate stripes may fail to be resolved as such, and under these circumstances the areas of different hue arise from true optical mixture. The hue assimilation persists, however, at viewing distances such that the overlay of stripes is clearly visible. In the composition illustrated in Figure 7 (Seitz, 1965), Anuszkiewicz handles a similar theme in a similar way, but with dots rather than lines. The red background is uniform throughout, but the appearance is one of sharply delimited and discontinuous areas of different hue. The separation into areas of different hue comes about through the superposition of blue, green, or yellow dots, and the work is appropriately called *All Things Do Live in the Three*. The dimensions of the original work are such that failures of optical resolution, and thus true optical mixture, may begin to occur at viewing distances beyond ten feet or so. But again the effect persists where the individual dots are quite clearly visible as such.

Assimilation effects are a major focus in some of Bridget Riley's paintings (de Sausmarez, 1970), where they sometimes show up as mysterious hue tonings in the whites of her swirling line patterns, only to disappear on close inspection.

What, then, is happening in the eye when we have colors that shift toward each other as if mixing, despite the fact that they also remain quite separate enough to delineate discrete forms? Clearly it seems that we must take another look at the

7 Richard Anuszkiewicz, *All Things Do Live in the Three*. Spatial dimensions and repeated alternation of elements give rise to assimilation rather than contrast. The original figure is executed in three different colors.

spatial organization of the retina, described earlier in this paper as a physiological mechanism ideally organized to yield color contrast, rather than mixture, effects. Figure 8 illustrates again, in the upper section, the same neural unit organization diagrammed in Figure 5. In the center we have represented the region of the retina that feeds excitatory impulses into this unit. If the retinal light image is of such fine grain that multiple different individual light points all fall within this one region, the unit will have no way of knowing that they are discrete light points, and it will respond as if the points had been perfectly superimposed, as in true light mixture. And the same will be true of another unit of this sort whose receptive field is centered right next to this one, and so on across the retina. With increasing image grain size, such units will be able to report "contour." If the retinal surface and the receptive fields of all its ganglion cells were perfectly uniform, that would be the end of the matter. But it is very important that we now remember that the retinal surface is not uniform; it has been estimated that the average size of the receptive field centers may increase by about sixfold or more from the center of the fovea to about twelve degrees away

Jameson
& Hurvich

(Hubel & Wiesel, 1960; Thomas, 1970). (Twelve degrees is equivalent to about seven feet in extent viewed at a distance of twenty feet.) It is also true that when electrical recordings are obtained from cells whose receptive fields are centered very close to each other in the same part of the retina, the receptive field centers are by no means identical in width (Hubel & Wiesel, 1960). What this means for perception is that, for a given repetitive pattern of lines imaged on the retina, an assembly of neural units like the one illustrated in the upper part of Figure 8 can be reporting that there is a line pattern present, and simultaneously, another assembly of more broadly receptive neural units, like the one illustrated in the lower part of the figure, can be reporting on the mixture of these lines with their adjacent image areas. So what we are proposing is that assimilation effects can occur because of parallel spatial processing in the visual system, just as color vision can occur because of parallel quality processing.

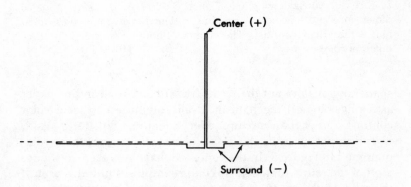

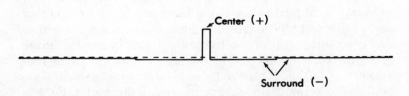

8   Like Figure 5, but represents response patterns of two different cells, the lower one having a larger spread of its receptive field on the retina than the upper one.

The kind of parallel processing that permits lightness and hue blending along with spatial resolution and good contour discrimination accounts for a special kind of visual interest that emerges in certain works of art. The interest derives from emergent perceptual effects that vary with the spatial dimensions of the image formed on the retina relative to its nonhomogeneous dimensional organization. Thus these particular effects in a painting or graphic work are more than usually dependent on the distance from which the work is viewed. To walk toward and back away from Seurat's *Grande Jatte*, for example, is also to experience an intriguing change in the dynamic quality of the painting. From afar, it may be a very quiet, static scene; very close, it can be a study in technique with the interest of an abstraction. But at a critical range of intermediate viewing distances, the variegated grain of the pigment tends to reach the threshold of resolution without breaking up the overall color composition, and to do so in different parts of the painting, depending on where one's line of regard is focused. It is at such a viewing distance that the liveliness of real outdoor light in a real outdoor scene is conveyed to the attentive viewer.

Although assimilation effects may strike one as part of the subject matter in the abstract and geometrical works of Anuszkiewicz and Riley, the techniques that depend on this property of the visual system are hardly new. They have been utilized for centuries in the graphic arts, and with masterly effect when in the hands of master artists. Consider the detail of an etching or woodcut in which the shading depends on hatching: the white of the background paper blends with the black of the hatching to yield the shades of the composition. If this were a matter of optical mixture, the structure or form of the hatching would make little difference, since it would not be resolved as such. But it is precisely because it is resolved that what Panofsky (1943) calls the "dynamic calligraphy" of a master print is so vital to the perceived effect. It is particularly Dürer's use of hatching lines—made variable in length and width and moved in curves so as to express form as well as light and shade—that Panofsky considers a major advance in Dürer's development as a superb graphic artist. As the intricacies of the visual system are systematically explored in laboratories of physiology and psychology, their understanding not only penetrates some of the mysteries of visual perception, but also sheds light on the creative works of our own time and throughout the history of art.

REFERENCES   Albers, J. *Interaction of color*. New Haven: Yale University Press, 1963.

Beck, J. *Surface color perception*. Ithaca and London: Cornell University Press, 1972.

Békésy, G. von. Mach- and Hering-type lateral inhibition in vision. *Vision Research 8* (1968): 1483–1499.

Bezold, W. von. *The theory of color in its relation to art and art-industry*. Boston: Prang, 1876. (S. R. Koehler, trans.)

de Sausmarez, M. *Bridget Riley*. Greenwich, Connecticut: New York Graphic Society, 1970.

DeValois, R. L. Central mechanisms of color vision. In R. Jung (Ed.), *Handbook of sensory physiology*. Vol. VII/3, *Central processing of visual information A: Integrative functions and comparative data*. Berlin: Springer, 1973.

Dowling, J. E., & Boycott, B. B. Organization of the primate retina: Electron microscopy. *Proceedings of the Royal Society* (London) *166B* (1966): 80–111.

Evans, R. M. *An introduction to color*. New York: Wiley, 1944.

Hubel, D. H., & Wiesel, T. N. Receptive fields of optic nerve fibers in the spider monkey. *Journal of Physiology* (London), *154* (1960): 572–580.

Hurvich, L. M., & Jameson, D. An opponent-process theory of color vision. *Psychological Review 64* (1957): 384–404.

Jameson, D., & Hurvich, L. M. Complexities of perceived brightness. *Science 133* (1961): 174–179.

Jameson, D., & Hurvich, L. M. Theory of brightness and color contrast in human vision. *Vision Research 4* (1964): 135–154.

Panofsky, E. *Albrecht Dürer*. Princeton, N. J.: Princeton University Press, 1943.

Polyak, S. L. *The retina*. Chicago: University of Chicago Press, 1941.

Ratliff, F. *Mach bands: Quantitative studies on neural networks in the retina*. San Francisco: Holden-Day, 1965.

Seitz, W. C. *The responsive eye*. New York: Museum of Modern Art, 1965.

Stevens, S. S. To honor Fechner and repeal his law. *Science 133* (1961): 80–86.

Thomas, J. P. Model of the function of receptive fields in human vision. *Psychological Review 77* (1970): 121–134.

Vasarely, V. *Vasarely II*. Neuchâtel: Éditions du Griffon, 1970 (H. Chevalier, trans.).

Wallach, H. Brightness constancy and the nature of achromatic colors. *Journal of Experimental Psychology 38* (1948): 310–324.

Hans Wallach

The Apparent Rotation of Pictorial Scenes

It is often noticed that the head of a portrait appears to turn when one walks past the picture. This apparent turning is even more impressive in the case of a landscape that shows strong perspective depth. The latter phenomenon has attracted little attention only because, for obvious reasons, such landscapes are rather rare. I noticed it first many years ago when walking past a landscape by Theodore Rousseau in the Frick Collection. It shows a country road flanked by rows of trees leading straight into the distance. When one walks past it the whole scene appears to turn, the foreground moving with the observer. This rotation direction is the same as the portrait head's, which appears to turn as if to look after the passing viewer.

The explanation of this phenomenon is connected with a rather recent development in the psychology of perception. When we move about, our environment is perceived as stable, although our movements cause a variety of sensory changes. The retinal projection of a scene we approach expands; when we turn the head, say, to the right, the environment shifts to the left relative to the eyes, which therefore receive the same stimulation as would be caused by a motion of the whole environment to the left; and there are other such phenomena. That these sensory changes do not cause the corresponding experiences of object growth and of motion of the visual field had earlier been ascribed to a tendency toward stability and rigidity of the experienced environment. But it now turns out that the nervous system deals piecemeal with each of these sensory changes. We do not see the environment move to the left when we turn the head to the right because of a nervous process that matches up kinesthetic information about the turning of the head with the visual change caused by the head movement. So accurate is this process that when one contrives, during a turning of the head, to have an artificial environment shift as little as 5 percent less 65 than normal, most observers will see the environment move, whereas the normal shift gives rise to an environment perceived as stationary (Wallach & Kravitz, 1965). Moreover, there is now evidence that the expansion of the projection of an approached scene does not cause the perception of a corresponding expansion precisely for the reason that this expansion occurs during one's forward movement.

The apparent rotation of a pictorial scene, when it is viewed successively from different directions, turns out to be a manifestation of a process that prevents still another sensory change caused by body movements from resulting in a perceptual change. When one moves forward, real objects that lie to the side of one's path are seen successively from different directions. It is easy to see that this produces the same stimulation that would be caused by a turning of the object when the eyes are stationary. The rotation of an object, too, causes one to see it successively from different directions. The two cases are the same as far as vision is concerned: Relative to one's eyes, a stationary object that lies to the side of one's movement path undergoes a partial rotation. This rotation or that of a whole scene that is viewed from a moving vantage point is hardly ever perceived. (An exception is the apparent rotation of a flat landscape observed from the window of a fast moving train.) Again this is not due to a general tendency to perceive a rigid environment; rather, it is the result of a special process that matches up the sensory change caused by the rotation of an object or a scene with information about one's changed vantage point. The existence of such a special process is best demonstrated by measuring its accuracy. This was done by finding out how much a luminous object in the dark may *actually* rotate as an observer moves past it without that turning being noticed. This work was done by Wallach, Stanton, and Becker (1974), who constructed an apparatus with which the object in question could be made to turn as the observer moved past it. The rate of this rotation in relation to the change in the observer's vantage point could be varied, and either turning direction relative to the observer's progress could be presented. As the observer walked back and forth past the object, its rotation rate was raised in small steps until the observer reported seeing the object turn.

With 44 observers tested, it was found that the object had to rotate, on the average, by 40.5 percent of the observer's change in position for that rotation to be reported reliably. Observers varied widely in their ability to detect the real object rotations that were made to take place as they moved past the object. Individual differences ranged from 12 to 63 percent of the position change when the object actually turned in the direction with the observer's progress, that is, clockwise when the object was on the observer's right.

To be sure, the matching-up process that underlies this performance is not as accurate by far as the one that keeps the visual environment from moving during a turning of the head. If it were completely accurate, an object would have to be entirely stationary as the observer moves past it to be so perceived: the slightest objective rotation would be detected. If it were as accurate as the matching-up process that keeps the visual environment from appearing to move when one turns one's head, an object that one passes would be perceived to turn when it actually turned only by 5 percent of the optical rotation that a stationary object undergoes relative to the moving eye. What was found is that the object must actually turn nearly 40 percent of that optical rotation for this turning to be perceived by the passing observer.

But this matching-up process is still accurate enough to account for the apparent rotation of a portrait as the viewer walks by. The painted head does not rotate at all in relation to the passing observer; being flat on the canvas, it cannot be seen from different directions. The moving observer sees the portrait always from the same direction. For a real head not to rotate optically in relation to the moving eye, it would have to turn objectively so that it is always seen from the same direction. In other words, it would have to rotate by 100 percent of the observer's position change, and this is, in close approximation, what the painted head does optically when the observer walks by. According to the measurements just reported, a rotation rate of 100 percent would cause rotation to be perceived by every one of the 44 observers, and that explains what happens in the picture gallery.

The same analysis applies to the painted landscape; here, too, whatever depth is *seen* in the picture, the lines that represent it lie on the picture surface. The length of the projections of these lines at the passing observer's eyes changes very little, at least, for those changes in his position during which he would normally look at a picture. The landscape, too, is viewed always from the same direction, which again is equivalent to a rotation of the scene by 100 percent of the observer's change in position.

So it turns out that the apparent rotation of a pictorial scene is a manifestation of the very process that prevents perceived rotation of real three-dimensional scenes which one passes. This process is probably learned. There is good evidence that another process that serves to keep the environment stable when we move is learned—that which prevents us from seeing the visual environment shift around us when we turn our head. That process can be altered in hours or even minutes, for instance by wearing spectacles that change the rate at which the visual environment is being displaced relative to the eyes during the turning of the head (Wallach & Kravitz, 1965). Initially such spectacles cause one to see the environment swing sideways during each head turning. This swinging diminishes gradually and, when the spectacles are taken off, a swinging in the direction opposite to that caused by the spectacles is observed during head turning. This effect will quickly subside until vision during head turning is again normal. These rapid alterations of the process that matches up information about the head turning with the sensory changes caused by it argue that the process had been learned in the first place.

It is probably not feasible to make an analogous demonstration for the process that prevents perception of the rotation of a real three-dimensional scene when one passes it. The matching up between one's position change and the object rotation that results from it is probably not accurate enough to obtain a process alteration that is measurable. It is, however, likely that the same principle operates in the development of the process that prevents the perception of rotation of a passed scene and of the process that keeps the perceived environment still during head movements. Since it is the turning of the head that causes the shifting of the environment, there is a strict covariance between the sensations produced by the shifting of the environment and the processes that represent the head movements in the nervous system. This is true of all visual sensory changes that are indirectly caused by our own movements: they are covariant with the sensations by which these body movements are represented. The sensory changes caused by the rotation of a passed scene and the sensations of movement involved in the observer's position change are similarly covariant. I believe that it is the covariance between the sensations of body movements and the visual sensory change that causes the development of the processes that here prevent the visual changes from having their normal effects in perception, such as seeing the environment move when it is displaced relative to the head or seeing a scene turn when, relative to the eyes, it undergoes a partial rotation. The view that a general principle is here in operation is supported by experiments in which, by artificial means, body movements are made to cause covariant sensory changes not normally produced by these movements. After prolonged exposure to these conditions, the perceptual experiences caused by these sensory changes will gradually subside.

REFERENCES

Wallach, H., & Kravitz, J. H. The measurement of the constancy of visual direction and of its adaptation. *Psychonomic Science 2* (1965): 217–218.

Wallach, H., Stanton, L., & Becker, D. The compensation for movement produced changes in object orientation. *Perception & Psychophysics 15* (1974): 339-343.

Hans
Wallach

69

James J. Gibson, George A. Kaplan, Horace N. Reynolds, Jr., and Kirk Wheeler

The Change from Visible to Invisible: A Study of Optical Transitions

Gibson suggested (1957) that *physical* motions, the motions of material objects, should be distinguished sharply from the corresponding *optical* motions that make them perceptible to an O. Several kinds and variables of optical motions were described, all of which were loosely termed "optical transformations," and these were illustrated in a motion picture film (Gibson, 1955).

We have recently been concerned, however, with another class of events, the perception of which needs to be understood. When an object *disappears from sight*, how is this event perceived and what is the optical basis for the perception? The question, far from having an obvious answer, is puzzling. The present study attempts to give an answer. It is illustrated by another motion picture film, a sequel to the first.

The term *disappearance* means a change from visible to invisible and the opposite term *appearance* means a change from invisible to visible. But this pair of terms is ambiguous, for there are two quite different kinds of events to which it may refer, that is, two ways in which an object may disappear and appear. It may *go out of sight* or *come into sight*, on the one hand, and it may *go out of existence* or *come into existence* on the other. The two cases are profoundly different, and human or animal Os clearly need

From *Perception and Psychophysics* 5 (1969): 113–116. Copyright 1969 by Psychonomic Journals, Inc. Reprinted by permission of the authors and publishers.

This essay is accompanied by a motion picture film with the same title referenced as Gibson, 1968 (Psychological Cinema Register, State College, Pa.). The production of the film over some four or five years was supported by the Office of Naval Research under Contract NONR 401(14) with Cornell University for research on the perception of motion and space.

to distinguish between the two cases if they are to cope with the permanent parts of their environment as contrasted with the impermanent parts—if they are to discriminate the persisting from the nonpersisting things. A thing that disappears merely because it is no longer projected by light to the O's point of view is not to be confused with a thing that disappears because it is no longer projected by light at all. The former can still be seen from another point of view; the latter cannot be seen from any point of view.

Note that an illuminated environment is being taken for granted in this discussion. We are not here considering the disappearance and appearance of *light,* or the sensation of light. We are talking about the disappearance and appearance of a material *surface* in the *presence* of light, that is, a perception. The theoretical distinction between sensation and perception has been elaborated by Gibson (1966). We are assuming that the disappearance of the whole environment with the absence of illumination and the reappearance of the whole environment with the presence of illumination is quite another problem than that of the disappearance and reappearance of a *part* of the environment, the whole of which is unaltered. The latter problem only is our present concern.

The question becomes, therefore, whether or not in the changing array of light to a point of observation there is a distinct kind of stimulus information for the perception of something that goes out of and comes into *sight* and another for the perception of something that goes out of and comes into *existence.* If the optical transitions are different in the two cases, and perhaps in their subtypes, a new perceptual theory is needed. We do not face the difficulties of the traditional explanations of how animals and children learn to *form concepts* of permanent things (e.g., Piaget, 1929), but we must explain how animals and children learn to *distinguish* between permanent and impermanent parts of the environment.

This new formulation of the problems that arise from the facts of visibility and invisibility owes much to the experimental work of Michotte (e.g., Michotte, Thines, & Crabbé, 1964). But there is an essential difference inasmuch as we consider the possibility of available stimulus information for the types of object disappearance and Michotte did not.

1 Going out of Sight and Coming into Sight

Consider the first case. A part of the environment, or a detachable object, may go out of sight because (a) it is hidden by another part of the environment, or (b) because it is hidden by another part of itself, or (c) because it becomes so distant from the point of observation that it "vanishes." The last subcase implies a level terrain that is unobscured out to the horizon; the first two subcases imply the existence of an *edge*. The event of becoming hidden by an edge results from straight-line projection in the light that fills an illuminated space, that is, from the fact that, for a given station point, some illuminated surfaces of the total layout are projected to it and others are unprojected. Some of them "face" the station point and others do not. We have various words for becoming hidden like *covering* and *screening* but the best word for it is *occlusion*. Optical occlusion deserves much more study than it has ever received in perspective geometry. As for the third subcase, the object that vanishes because its distance becomes too great, it is also a consequence of the geometrical laws of perspective projection but it does not involve edge-occlusion; it involves the "vanishing point" of perspective and the "horizon" of the earth, or the principle of what will be called optical minification.

Occlusion, then, entails one thing in front of another, or one surface in front of another, with reference to a point of observation. It has been called interposition or "superposition" in the literature of pictorial depth-perception. But actually *change* of occlusion is what occurs in life as objects move and as Os move about in the world. Stationary occlusion as represented in a picture or a frozen optic array has been studied by perceptionists but change of occlusion has not.

Vanishing into a point does not entail the relation in-front-of (or behind) but it has been studied and puzzled about for centuries. The kinetic fact that the projection of an object shrinks to a point as its distance increases, and the stationary fact that parallel lines on the earth are projected as lines that converge to a point on the horizon are at the very heart of our conception of abstract space.

It is important to note that, in all three subcases, going out of sight is reciprocal to coming into sight; one is simply the inverse of the other. The motion of an object that makes it disappear always has an opposite that makes it reappear; similarly, the

Gibson
et al.

locomotion of an O that makes anything disappear can always be reversed so as to make it reappear.

2 Going out of Existence and Coming into Existence

Consider next the second case. When an object or part of the environment ceases to "exist," the fact is that its physical state has been changed by disintegration, solution, evaporation, sublimation, combustion, or dissipation. The surface that reflected light has ceased to exist. To be sure, the atomic matter has not; the latter has been *conserved*, as the physicists say, although its structure is altered. Nevertheless, even if matter cannot be annihilated, a light-reflecting surface can.

Conversely, an object can come into existence by crystallization or coagulation or condensation or sedimentation or, at a higher level of chemistry, by cell-growth. When it does, it begins to reflect light and becomes visible. But note that these processes by which an entity comes into visible existence are not simple reversals or opposites of the processes by which it goes out of visible existence, as are the motions and locomotions of the first case. The processes of dissolution and biological death are usually irreversible. This fact is connected with what the physicists call *entropy*.

We are now prepared to study the optical transitions that arise from these different events. What are the changes in the optic array at a point of observation that can be distinguished by an O?

1A Progressive Covering and Uncovering

When the edge of one surface conceals or reveals another surface in the world, what happens in the structure of the optic array? What happens optically seems to be as follows. The adjacent units of optical texture on one side of a possible division in the optic array are preserved while adjacent units of optical texture on the other side of the division are progressively added to the array (uncovering) or are progressively subtracted from the array (covering). The *decrementing* of texture corresponds to a surface being concealed while the *incrementing* of texture corresponds to a surface being revealed. That side of the dividing line on which there is deletion or accretion always corresponds to the surface that is *behind*; that side on which there is neither always corresponds to the surface that is *in front* (Kaplan, 1968). Gibson (1966, p. 203) called this optical transition "wiping and unwiping" but these terms are metaphorical and are not mathematically precise. An effort to formalize the above rule is given in the appendix to this paper.

Note that this formula says nothing about the absolute *motion* (transposition) of objects in the world or of the O's position in the world, nor does it say anything about the absolute motion of the elements of optical texture in the array. Progressive deletion of texture can result from either a rightward motion of the covering surface or a leftward motion of the covered surface; progressive accretion can result from either a leftward motion of the covering surface or a rightward motion of the covered surface; in short, a thing can be *covered* by either of two physical motions. The special case of an object that moves behind a stationary occluding edge is only one case. It has attracted attention because of the paradoxical fact that the motion of the object continues to be "seen" after it is no longer projected in the optic array. Reynolds (1968) has verified this discovery of Michotte and has further investigated the experience of occluded motion.

When this optical transition of progressive accretion or deletion is experimentally produced by a motion picture display, an occluding edge is in fact perceived by an O, although the display consists only of a random texture divided into two parts. When the incrementing or decrementing of texture ceases, the edge is no longer perceived and a continuous textured surface is seen instead (Gibson, 1968). These facts cannot be illustrated with a stationary picture; the reader should view the film if possible. The diagram given in the appendix, however, may be of help in visualizing the phenomena.

1B   The Conversion of a Surface into an Edge

A "movable" object in the environment is one that is detached from the permanent layout of the environment. Such an object, if opaque, occludes not only a part of the environment (the "ground" or "background") but also a part of itself, namely its "back" surface as distinguished from its "front" surface. Considering a polyhedron (an object with plane surfaces that face in different directions) we can assert that when it is rotated (or when an O moves around it) a *front* face is converted into a *back* face. As the slant angle of the front face increases the perspective projection of its form and texture is increasingly transformed; the transformation is loosely called "foreshortening" and its limit is a geometrical line. The optical figure and its components are compressed, as it were, along one dimension only. Meanwhile, of course, the slant angle of another face of the object *decreases,* its form and texture undergoing the reverse transformation.

A motion picture display of this optical transition does indeed yield the perception of a surface that is seen to turn until it passes through the position of "edge-on." (A randomly textured cube was employed, but another polyhedron would have served.) The surface no longer *faces* the O but it persists phenomenally as a face of the object that has gone out of sight (Gibson, 1968). When the sequence is reversed by running the film backward, a perfectly normal perception occurs of a surface that has *come into* sight.

1c *The Vanishing of a Surface into the Distance*

When an object progressively becomes more distant from the point of observation, its counterpart in the optic array shrinks, and the limit of this contraction is a geometrical point. If the object is in the sky or on level terrain it will not be occluded or hidden but it will nevertheless vanish by "minification." The figure corresponding to the front face of the object undergoes a size-transformation, all ratios or proportions in the figure being preserved until its visual angle becomes zero. The reverse transformation occurs when an object becomes progressively closer to the point of observation.

When this optical change is displayed on a motion picture screen the percept is of something that goes out of sight into the distance. This fact has been exploited in animated cartoon films. When Mickey Mouse is seen to zoom off at enormous speed he disappears without ceasing to exist. With magnification, similarly, a percept results of something coming out of the distance, that is, of approach. This can be simulated with a point-source shadow-projector (Gibson, 1957) and the method has been used by Schiff (1965) to investigate the reactions of animals to the information for approach.

In conclusion, there do seem to be specific optical transitions corresponding to these three types of the events called *going out of sight* and *coming into sight.* Moreover, there is some evidence to show that animals and children distinguish the transitions and perceive the corresponding events. It should now be possible to carry out formal experiments with animals and children at various stages of development. Some research with human infants confronted with progressive occlusion and disocclusion of an object has been reported by Bower (1967) but the rationale of these experiments is not the same as that of our demonstrations.

We now turn to the events called *going out of existence* and *coming into existence*. The corresponding optical transitions are more complex and are not so easily described. An attempt will be made, however, to specify three examples that can be displayed on a motion picture screen.

2A *Evaporation and Sublimation*

When a puddle of water evaporates or a chunk of solid carbon dioxide sublimates, the projected contour in the optic array shrinks and the optical texture within the contour changes, but in a way quite unlike the shrinkage and change that occur with optical contraction or minification. The figure shrinks irregularly, the texture does not become more dense, and ratios do not remain invariant. Phenomenally, the object is seen to disappear but it is *not* seen to vanish into the distance.

A motion picture display of a piece of "dry ice" disintegrating against a dark background yields the perception of something that ceases to exist. When the sequence is reversed in temporal order by running the film backward, the perception is "strange." There is then a suggestion of *growth* and of a substance that increases in size but this is not the same as the optical magnification that corresponds to the approach of an object out of the distance.

2B *Fading Away by Increasing Transparency*

The mythical conception of ghosts or spirits, expressed in the Platonic conception of form without substance, has sometimes included the assumption that an opaque reflecting surface can become transparent, like one of water or glass, and can then become wholly nonreflecting, like air itself. This event does not actually occur but some men have believed that it could. It is inaccurately called "dematerialization" by believers in spirits, the opposite process being "materialization." A discussion of the optics of transparency is offered by Gibson (1966, p. 216).

The optical information for this hypothetical event can be produced by the method of double-exposing photographic film, and it is often used in the motion picture transition termed a "dissolve." Occasionally it has been used in cinematography to yield the illusion of an object or a man becoming a ghost.

A motion picture display can be made beginning with a textured rectangle on a differently textured background, progressing to a mixture of the texture of the background with that of the rectangle, and ending with the texture of the background only. The O of this display perceives a rectangular object that goes out of existence. He does not report that it goes into the distance, or is hidden, or turned away. The opposite transition yields an experience of coming into existence, and it is even more anomalous.

2c *Being Consumed by Eating*

Of all the kinds of substantial objects in the environment one of the most attractive is that of food objects. They are discriminated at an early stage of development and are further differentiated throughout life. They are peculiar, however, in being relatively impermanent; they disappear when they are eaten. One subclass of human food objects disappears from the optic array in successive "bites."

A motion picture sequence has been made beginning with a white disk on a black ground, with curved segments of the disk being successively deleted (cut out) from the periphery inward. This optical transition is different from the *continuous progressive* deletion of adjacent texture elements that corresponds to occlusion of an object. Os of this display are unanimous in perceiving a cookie or its equivalent that is being *eaten up*. The object is clearly seen to go out of existence. It is possible that even young children will perceive the same event with this display if they have come to notice that the successive deleting of curved parts of a figure corresponds to something being eaten. When the sequence is reversed in temporal order, another quite different event is perceived, but it is very "strange" for the adult Os and it would probably also prove to be so for the child.

The three transitions described above do not exhaust the possibilities. (We have not yet attempted to simulate the optics of melting or crumbling or breaking, although it could probably be done.) Nevertheless, a tentative conclusion would be that the two general ways in which an object can disappear are easily distinguished, and that they are distinguishable on the basis of optical stimulus information. Something that goes out of sight but continues to exist is not confused with something that disappears because it ceases to exist.

Discussion

It has long been taken for granted by developmental psychologists and philosophers of perception that the young child differs from the adult in the following respect: he cannot help believing that something which goes out of sight ceases to exist (Piaget, 1929). This follows from the theory of sensation-based perception, that is, from the assumption that when the sensation ceases the perception must cease, and the further assumption that imagination can take the place of sensation. But it now seems very doubtful that a young child has the belief that whatever goes out of sight ceases to exist. His perceptions are probably not based on his fleeting sensations but on the visual pickup of optical information. His perceptions are in Michotte's term "amodal" (Michotte, Thines, & Crabbé, 1964). When the optical information is of one general sort the persistence of an object is specified; when it is of another general sort the nonpersistence of the object is specified. All the child has to do is distinguish the two general cases. Developmentally, he may have to learn to distinguish them but the development is one of perception, not of belief.

The optical transitions described in this paper, and displayed in the accompanying film, are of two general types. One is a *reversing* transition and the other is not. All of the reversing transitions looked equally natural whether the film was run forward or backward; the others did not look natural when the film was run backward. The reversing optical transitions are caused by motions of the object and by movements of the O from one place to another; the nonreversing optical transitions are caused by the destruction or creation of the reflecting surfaces that constitute an object. There are mathematical properties of the reversing transitions to specify the temporal existence of the object, both preexistence and postexistence; the properties of the nonreversing transitions specify either the going out of existence or the coming into existence of the object.

In his experimental studies of the "screening effect" and the "tunnel effect" with moving visual forms, Michotte confronted a paradox: the fact of the phenomenal persistence of an object after it had been occluded by an edge. On the traditional assumption that the sensation of an object, the color patch in the visual field, is entailed in its perception, a nonpersisting sensation *cannot* yield a persisting perception. An occluded object ought to be indistinguishable from a destroyed object, whereas it is in fact distinguishable. A radical resolution of the paradox is to assume that the sensation of an object is *not* entailed in its perception; all that is required for perception is the colorless and formless information to specify a persisting object on the one hand or a destroyed object on the other.

APPENDIX   *The Hypothesis of Deletion/Accretion for Edge Perception*

Consider the following string of symbols:

12345FGHIJ.

They are intended to stand for adjacent elements of optical texture across an *optic array*. The nature of these "elements" is unspecified and the absolute locations are unspecified; they are simply adjacent. The numerals and the letters do not necessarily stand for two kinds of elements; they only imply that the array is divisible into two parts.

1. If the elements 12345 are preserved and the elements FGHIJ are progressively deleted from the array in the order FGH . . . , an occluding surface is specified by the numerals and an occluded surface by the letters; an edge is specified at Element 5, and depth is to the *right*.

2. If the elements FGHIJ are preserved and the elements 12345 are progressively deleted in the order 543 . . . , an occluding surface is specified by the letters and an occluded surface by the numerals; an edge is specified at Element F, and depth is to the *left*.

3. If the elements FGHIJ are preserved and the elements 12345 are progressively *accreted* in the order 678 . . . , an occluding surface is specified by the letters and an occluded surface by the numerals; an edge is specified at Element F, and depth is to the *left*.

4. If the elements 12345 are preserved and the elements FGHIJ are progressively *accreted* in the order EDC . . . , an occluding surface is specified by the numerals and an occluded surface by the letters; an edge is specified at Element 5, and depth is to the *right*.

Hence the part of the array that suffers deletion or accretion corresponds to a surface that is *behind* and is being concealed or revealed. The part of the array that is preserved corresponds to a surface that is *in front* and is concealing or revealing. The terminal element of the array that is preserved corresponds to the *edge*. A test of this hypothesis has been carried out by Kaplan (1968), along with another hypothesis dealing with the impression of mere depth-at-an-edge without the impression of one surface existing behind another.

REFERENCES

Bower, T. G. R. The development of object-permanence: Some studies of existence constancy. *Perception & Psychophysics* 2 (1967): 411–418.

Gibson, J. J. *Optical motions and transformations as stimuli for visual perception*. Motion picture film. Psychological Cinema Register, State College, Pa., 1955.

Gibson, J. J. Optical motions and transformations as stimuli for visual perception. *Psychological Review,* 64 (1957): 288–295.

Gibson, J. J. *The senses considered as perceptual systems*. Boston: Houghton Mifflin, 1966.

Gibson, J. J. *The change from visible to invisible: A study of optical transitions*. Motion picture film. Psychological Cinema Register, State College, Pa., 1968.

Kaplan, G. A. Kinetic disruption of optical texture: The perception of depth at an edge. Cornell doctoral dissertation, 1968.

Michotte, A., Thines, G., & Crabbé, G. Les complements amodaux des structures perceptives. *Studia Psychologica*. Louvain: Publ. Univ. de Louvain, 1964.

Piaget, J. *The child's conception of the world*. New York: Harcourt Brace, 1929.

Reynolds, H. N. Temporal estimation in the perception of occluded motion. *Perceptual & Motor Skills* 26 (1968): 407–416.

Schiff, W. Perception of impending collision. *Psychological Monographs* (1965): 79 No. 604.

II
VISUAL THINKING

Although we may agree with Rudolf Arnheim that any distinction between visual perception and visual thinking is artificial, several studies in this part deal with art work in categories distinct from those usually employed in the experimental psychology of perception.

Schaefer-Simmern discusses children's drawings from early scribbling to increasingly clear and unitary use of visual form. The child's drawings are seen to parallel changes in his relation to his world, to reflect his efforts to grasp this world, and to reveal his insights into its objects; drawings reflect the child's inner psychological reality. The author sees in these drawings the beginnings of a visualized point of view—a point of view, he fears, that often succumbs to the rationalistic approach of our schools.

A very different kind of excursion into the past is made by Nash, whose photographs reveal patterns in Roman architecture for the most part visible only when a building has fallen into ruins. They point out a visual thinking in Roman architecture that is not superficially apparent.

Finally, Gardner reflects on an exhibition of forgeries that permitted a variety of kinds of comparison with the original works of art. The illuminating comparison, he concludes, provides a means of heightening aesthetic awareness or of promoting visual thinking. In connection with the exhibit, the role of language in artistic instruction is considered.

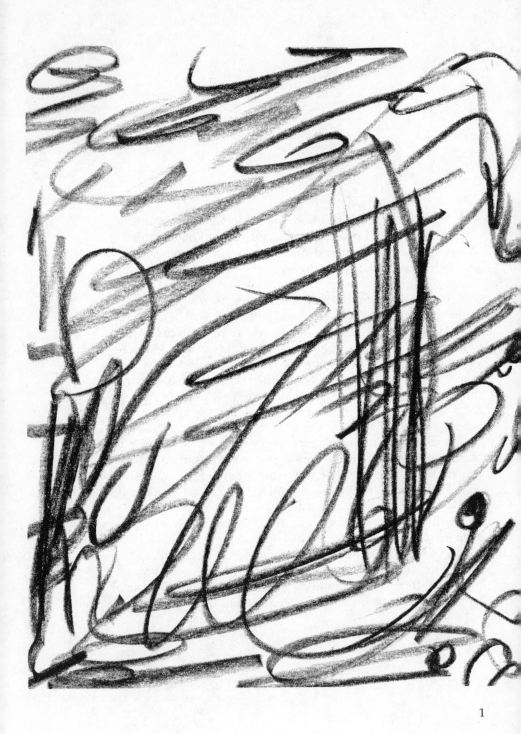

Henry Schaefer-Simmern

Basic Structures in the Earliest Beginnings of Artistic Activity

In the beginning of the child's and early man's pictorial activity, visual structures are revealed which are of basic importance in the building up of works of visual art.

What happens in the infant's mind when he first makes a mark on the surface of a paper? His expressive gestures, recorded by whatever means, even with a dirty finger, will certainly surprise him. Even more, he may become aware that a certain change has taken place on the paper's surface (Fig. 1). It may dawn on him that he himself has caused this change in the world outside himself. But by this self-caused change, the outside world becomes the child's world and has new meaning for him. No wonder, then, that this experience brings about a strong urge to repeat his actions over and over again. Can one see here the earliest roots of man's creative visualization, his need to realize his ideas pictorially and to transform the outside world into his own humanized world? It seems to me that this primary creative attitude finds its earliest realization in what is called "scribbling"—a term which, for the adult, usually signifies mere accidental disorder. I do not believe that the child in this stage of his mental development is aware that the outcome of his activity lacks order. He feels, rather, that he is involved in what we may describe as an imaginative visual wholeness.

With the child's gradually increasing observation of the outcome of his visual gestures, he seems to become aware of their complexity. He senses the need for a clearer visual grasping. The great variety of his visual markings begins to disappear and multiple, but simple, curved and vertical and horizontal line combinations begin to emerge. In other words, more concentrated and simpler structures evolve out of the previous visual composites (Figs. 2 and 3). These structures are no longer scattered over a particular surface; they tend rather to stand singly. Slowly they take on a certain compactness consisting of multiple 87 lines with simple relationships of direction holding their shapes together. This compactness is the result of rhythmical movements of up and down, right and left, and oval and circular gestures. Regardless of how clear or hazy these shapes may appear, they may already be considered as the very beginnings of primary figures. They can only exist visually, however, through their surrounding empty ground. It may seem naïve to suggest that very simple artistic structures may emerge at this early stage. Nevertheless, figure-ground and line relationships, no matter how simple, belong to the very foundation of artistic activity and production.

As a result of a basic human experience of the child, more accentuated figure-ground and line relationships develop. These will be visually recorded by the child since, with the sensation of being in the center of a certain space, which embraces the young child like a ground within which he is the figure, a physical and mental security is felt and expressed by the rotary movement of the body. This is a movement in which the child's self is the center from which he tends to unfold himself to the outside or return from the outside to the center. This is visually realized by a definite structure that is usually termed a spiral (Fig. 4). Every part of this structure, whether it started from the center or the outside, is determined by the curve just preceding it. This spiraling structure leads to a clearer total figure than the preceding

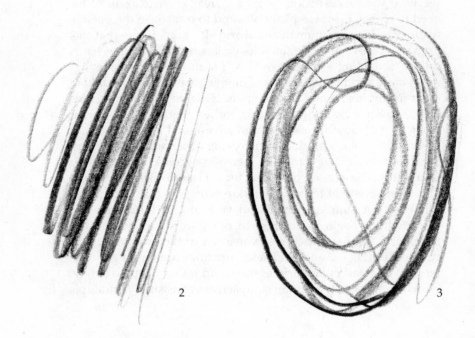

2   3

structures, which merely consisted of multiple lines. A primary, very simple, but organized whole is revealed. We have before us, therefore, a primitive example of Gestalt formation (*Gestaltung*).

In all early epochs, such distinct forms as the spiral have been endowed with sacred symbolic meaning. The spiral can be found at the end of the paleolithic era in France, as well as in the neolithic civilizations and the Bronze Age. In Egypt and China it stands for the flowing of life and of water; in other parts of the world it signifies coming and going, birth and death, as well as the thriving of life and the growing and unfolding of the universal spirit.

This sense of being in an all-embracing spatial surrounding, experienced and responded to by his rotary bodily movements, makes the child conscious of the world in which he exists and helps him to define his limits. In this way he gains a certain mental stability. The oscillating and curving quality of the spiral structure, repeated and observed by him again and again, cannot ultimately fulfill his creative needs. Gradually, therefore, the spiral lines become more and more reduced and give way to the creation of a simply outlined, evenly curved shape—a circular figure (Fig. 5). A definite and balanced figure, emerging from an empty surrounding, constitutes a clear and convincing figure-ground relationship. Such a figure indicates the establishment

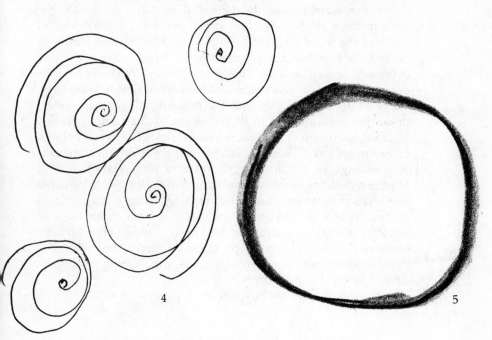

4   5

of a stable attitude, of equilibrium and security. From this moment in time the young child knows *where* he exists. He approaches both his surroundings and those things that enter his mind with a newly acquired consciousness of form. He can visually conceive all things in this most generalized way. To the child this structure represents the world he knows, and through this structure he brings that world within his grasp.

For long periods of time, prehistoric and early man shaped the essential parts of the world around him in terms of this primary form. Most prehistoric dwellings up to neolithic man, and those of today's indigenous tribes as well, are circular in shape. This simple structure adumbrates a solution to the basic mental problem of every genuine artist, the adoption of a visualized point of view with regard to the world around him. Both the circular figure and the spiral have, by means of their particular structure, achieved universal symbolic meaning. The circle, for example, becomes the basis of the mandala. Its form stands both for the idea of eternity and of the universe, for the all-embracing principle of divine manifestation, and for the final Absolute.

As we have already seen, at this primitive stage of development of visual conceiving, the circular figure stands symbolically for all things. Martha, a child of three years and five months, drew a picture of concentric circles (Fig. 6). She and her classmates were constantly reminded to draw slowly so that their pictures might look clear and "beautiful." When she had finished the inner circle in her drawing, Martha said loudly to herself, "Mama," and when making the larger outer circle, she expressed herself audibly, "has a new dress." What are the underlying formative facts in the achievement of this drawing? The shape of the inner circle, with the meaning of "Mama," determines the line direction of the outer circle: "has a new dress." The empty ground of the inner circle becomes the inside volume of the outer circle. Both together form a perfect early gestalt. Any change in the figure-ground and line relationship of Martha's drawing would disturb the total figure. Such a change would also be detrimental to the meaning, to the content of this picture. Thus it should be evident that in this very early stage of intuitive visual formation, a universal, fundamental artistic problem has already found a primitive solution—the indivisibility of content and form, with the content becoming totally absorbed by the artistic form.

John, a five-year-old boy, drew "A pond with fish" (Fig. 7).

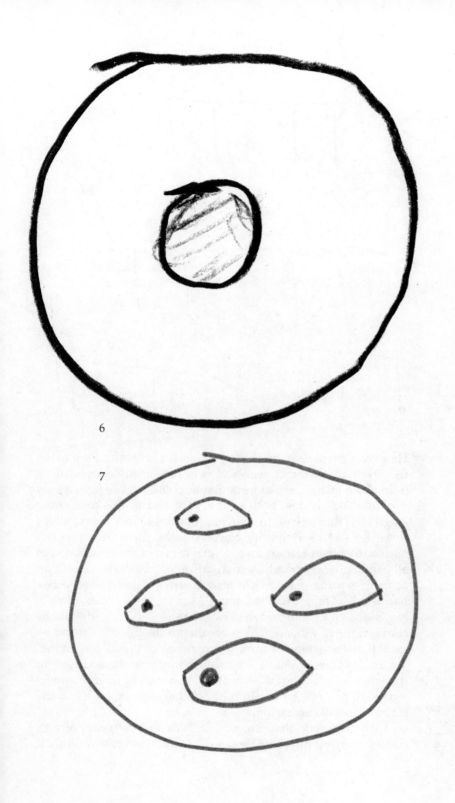

6

7

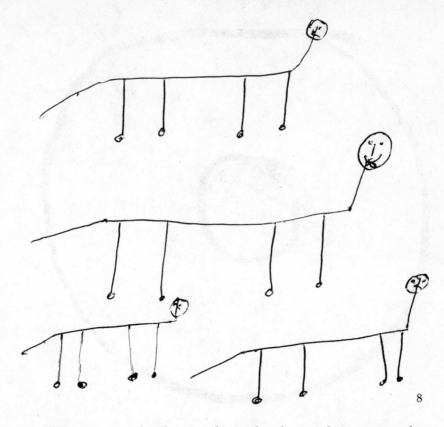

8

He gave a circular shape to the pool and an oval structure to the fish. He had obviously seen real fish, but his mind was still so dominated by the circular form that he could deviate from it only slightly. The shapes, both of the pool and of the fish, stand singly for themselves in primary figure-ground relationship. Regardless of its simplicity or complexity, the achievement of such a totality of form is an essential factor in the production of all genuine works of art. A comparison of this drawing with an actually existing pond might lead one to suppose that the boy had tried to reproduce the pond as seen from above, from a bird's-eye view. John, however, was conscious only of what he could conceive visually. His is an attempt to grasp *his* world by mental relationships of form in the realm of visual conceiving. We are confronted here with another fundamental analogue to the artistic attitude: art does not imitate nature but transforms it. Art does this by the creation of relationships of forms in the realm of visual conceiving.

Three different children, about three to four years of age, created the next pictures (Figs. 8–10). Both the figures and their

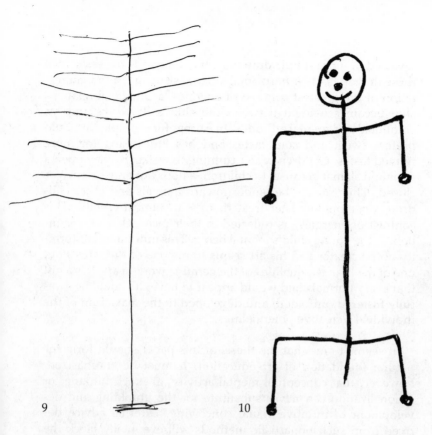

9   10

lines, represented singly, are brought out by the primary figure-ground relationship. In addition, each picture consists of a definite line relationship characterized by the greatest contrast of direction, the horizontal-vertical. In effect, each structure reveals a very early, but perfect, unity of form. But there is something of still more basic artistic importance in these beginnings. For instance, the structure of the tree shows that something has been observed going up (the trunk) and from this, something going out (branches). Similar observation of, and insight into, the structure of objects are recorded by the drawing of four dogs and by that of a man. The child comprehends intuitively and visually something of the essence of the things of his world, a mental attitude that is implicit in all works of art, but that has gradually disappeared because of the dominant development of conceptual thinking as the foundation of natural science and technology. Intuitive artistic vision is then replaced by conceptual knowledge, by the tyranny of rules of "how to do it." When this occurs, true intuitive artistic vision has been killed.

Still another essential characteristic of a genuine work of art is

Schaefer-
Simmern

93

revealed in these simple drawings. If one regards the essence of these drawings, their horizontal-vertical structure, as a manifestation of the greatest contrast of energies, a congenial relationship becomes evident between the child's drawings and his emotional and mental attitudes. In eating, for example, the child prefers sweet and sour tastes and has little liking for more refined tastes. Children prefer running to walking. They open a door and slam it because, to children, a door can only be open or closed. Children can be tender toward animals and other children, yet moments later treat them with utmost cruelty. This contrast of energies, as reflected in their pictorial works, symbolizes the young child's mental being. This innermost conformity of the creator and his art seems to me one of the rarest, but one of the highest, qualities of the genuine work of art. It is a gift that every normal child would appear to have. It should be carefully fostered, unfolded, and developed to the maximum of the individual's creative potentialities.

It seems to me that the thesis of this paper should form the natural foundation of art education. It must be emphasized, however, that conceptual mental activity, abstract thinking, or rationalization can never substitute for the unfolding and development of intuitive visual conceiving. External advice derived from such nonartistic methods will eventually block the natural growth of the child's artistic activity. It is generally accepted that the development of scientific thinking is the essential purpose of early education in the sciences. Since, however, as indicated in this short essay, basic artistic experience is already present in the work of young children, education in the arts should begin in the earliest school grades and should be continued on the basis of the natural laws of visual conceiving. Unfortunately, we are far from adopting such a view either of art or of education.

Ernest Nash

Hidden Visual Patterns in Roman Architecture and Ruins

Roman architecture is full of constructive and decorative patterns often so rigidly applied that certain patterns in brickwork make it possible to ascribe the construction to a given period. But not only did the builders create well-designed patterns; nature itself created patterns through the decay and final destruction of a building.

The public Roman thermae had huge halls for hot or lukewarm baths (*caldaria* and *tepidaria*); they were heated by hot air that was introduced from a furnace into a hollow space under a floor of square tiles measuring two feet, each supported at the corners by small brick columns or pillars. When such a hall was destroyed and the tiles of the floor had disappeared, the rows of little brick columns remained, forming a pattern which was not visible when the building was intact (Fig. 1).

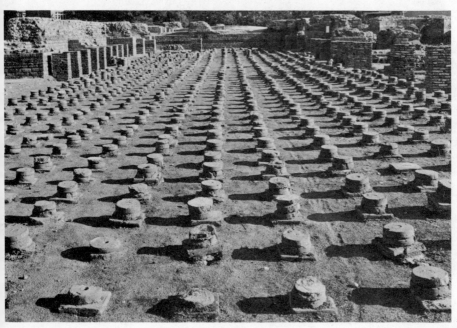

Another pattern, based on the building technique of Roman baths and created by the destruction of the building, derives from the heating system of a bathtub, in this instance in a private house at Magdalensberg in Austria (Fig. 2). The pattern consists of regular quadrangular holes surrounding the bathtub. Nothing of it was visible before the destruction of the bathroom. The heating of thermae, whether public or in private houses, was not restricted to the floors; the hollow area under the floors was extended to the walls by means of tubes made of hollow bricks, which were covered by plaster or marble revetting. Only when the walls were destroyed and the tubes cut to the level of the bathtub did the pattern of holes appear.

2

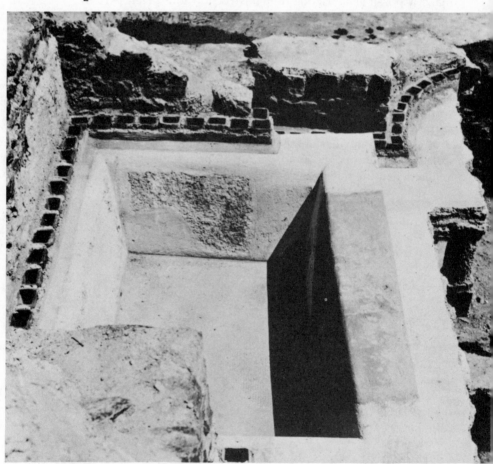

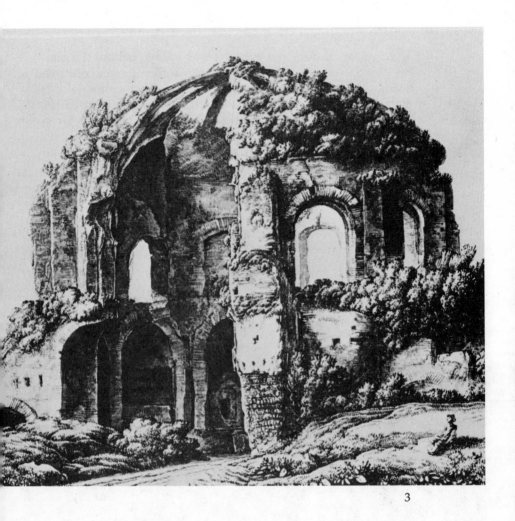

3

Another type of Roman construction, brick ribs forming the framework of vaulting, became visible as a result of the partial collapse of the dome of the so-called "Temple of Minerva Medica" near the railroad station "Termini" in Rome (Fig. 3). The ten-sided building was a pavilion in the gardens of the Emperor Gallienus dating from the middle of the third century A.D. When the dome covered the building nothing could be seen of the brick ribs, the intervening spaces being filled in with lightweight material. With the decay of the building, the filling material fell down and the framework of ten radiating ribs formed a pattern, as seen in this drawing from the end of the eighteenth century. In 1828 the pattern disappeared when the framework went the way of the rest of the dome.

Ernest
Nash

97

A wealth of designed patterns was hidden behind the plaster, stucco, or marble facing of Roman walls. Roman construction technique used bricks or small square tufa stones set in a diamond-shaped pattern, *opus reticulatum*, only as a curtain. The wall itself consisted of concrete made from rubble and mortar. A perfect curtain of variegated reticulate is represented by a cella wall of the Capitolium in Terracina (Fig. 4). This very exact pattern can still be seen all over the Roman world today. In ancient times it was almost always covered by wall facing, plaster, stucco, or marble plates.

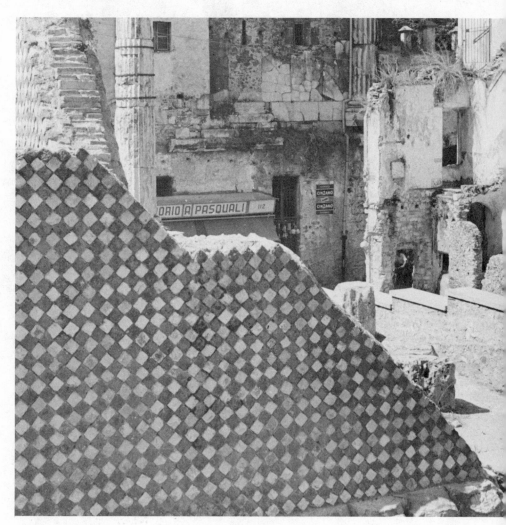

The "herring bone" pattern is limited to brick construction and mostly used as pavement in courtyards, shops and other commercial buildings, and squares. In a tomb of the necropolis of Isola Sacra between Ostia and Porto (Fiumicino), it is used as a vertical wall (Fig. 5); in contrast to the patterns discussed thus far, it was probably not covered with plaster.

The concrete walls on Rome's Via dei Fori Imperiali (Fig. 6) belonged to Nero's Golden House. The pattern of vertical lines is produced by the wooden form into which the concrete was poured, a technique still used in our day.

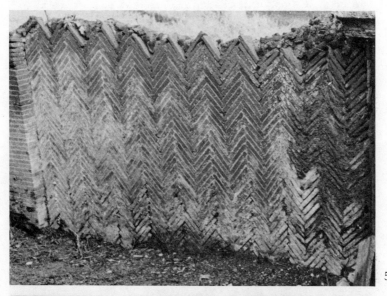

5

6

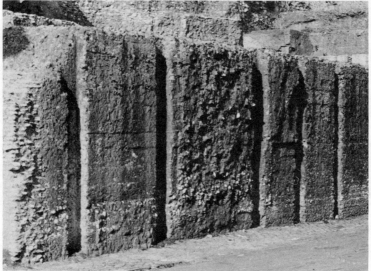

Ernest
Nash

99

65883

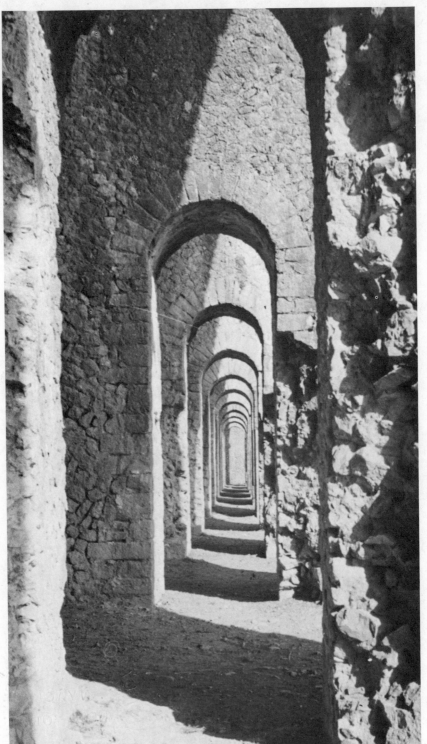

7

The Temple of Jupiter Anxur at Terracina stands on a large artificial terrace faced by impressive stone arches, behind which runs a 60 meter long passageway. The walls supporting the terrace are pierced by arched openings that form an architectural pattern, the perception of which is largely dependent on the point of view of the observer. Only when one stands in the exact center of the passageway does the perspective view of the arches become a pattern (Fig. 7).

Another primitive architectural pattern is formed by buttress blocks placed at regular intervals against the long side of a temple podium (Fig. 8). It was excavated on the Magdalensberg (Austria) in the Roman province of Noricum where, from the first century B.C., an important trading settlement had developed. The buttress blocks and the podium of the temple were once covered by marble.

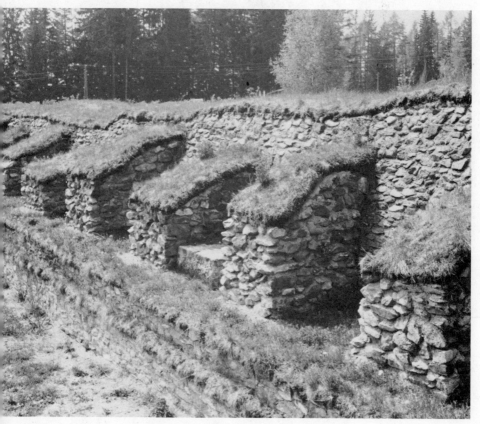

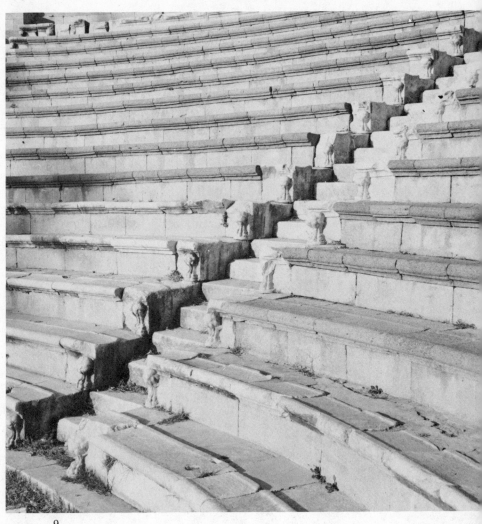

9

The well-preserved Roman theater in the Asklepieion at Pergamon (Turkey) suggested the pattern shown in the photograph
(Fig. 9). Needless to say, the semicircular auditorium of a theater
with its radially arranged stepways is a pattern in itself. The
photograph, however, shows a section of the auditorium, the
regular tiers of which are diagonally cut by one stepway. This
pattern is purely visual, created not by a decorative or functional
design, but by the viewpoint of the observer, deliberately limit-
ing the field of vision.

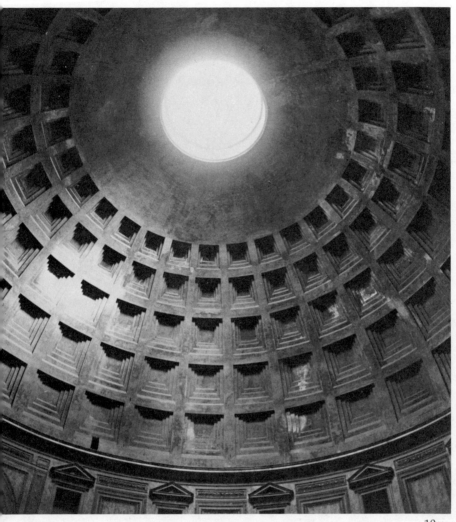

10

By contrast, the coffered dome of the Pantheon in Rome (Fig. 10) exposes a concentric and universal design which, seen from the ground, produces the same effect from every conceivable point of observation. The pattern of the stepped coffers is obviously designed to emphasize the perspective from the springing of the cupola to its open hole.

One might conclude that Roman architecture shows more "visual thinking" than appears on the surface.

Ernest Nash

Howard Gardner
Illuminating Comparisons in the Arts

During the summer of 1973, the Minneapolis Institute of Arts mounted an exhibit of several hundred works of art drawn from diverse persons and schools; included were representatives of several aesthetic media, ranging from paintings and drawings to book covers and pottery. The show was billed as an "educational exhibit." This struck me as a curious designation from one point of view, since a noneducational museum exhibit is difficult to envisage. And yet, as the exhibit lent itself superlatively to pedagogical purposes, perhaps the description is justified. I had the opportunity to attend the exhibit on a number of occasions; it proved a singularly entertaining and edifying aesthetic experience. In these paragraphs, I will seek to uncover the reasons for my positive reaction and consider whether some wider principles might be culled from this experience. Using the exhibit as a point of departure, I will examine the technique of the "illuminating comparison" as a means of heightening aesthetic awareness.

Fully half of the works on display in Minneapolis would normally have been a source of keen embarrassment to the curators and trustees of a museum. For the director and the curatorial staff had assembled a collection of "Fakes, Forgeries, and other Deceptions"; deceits of every variety were conveniently juxtaposed alongside the originals they were purporting to represent. By this happy arrangement, the viewer was granted the invaluable opportunity to compare and contrast originals and forgeries.

Unquestionably, such a collection constituted a veritable feast

This paper has been drawn in part from a report prepared for the Council on Museum Education and was supported in part by the National Institutes of Education, through grant NE-G-00-3-1069 to Harvard Project Zero.

for the connoisseur. Not only did he have the opportunity to examine works seldom on display, but he could also bring to bear varied tools of technical analysis, ranging from knowledge of the methods and materials available in different historical periods to details of the ways in which specific artists signed, dated, and otherwise incorporated distinctive marks onto canvases. Indeed a wide array of scholars and critics visited the Minneapolis show, delivered suitable lectures, praised its catalogues, and urged the preservation of the displays in one form or another.

Too often, however, exhibits are mounted just for the cognoscenti. The hypothetical average viewer may well feel alienated or abandoned by such professional tours de force. Lacking the necessary background and training in analytic procedures, the untrained observer cannot fully appreciate the rationale for the show, the significance of particular selections (and omissions), the technical language of the catalogue, and the intent and impact of this or that curatorial aside. At best, the typical gallery-goer may gain some pleasure from one or another work, or from the elegance with which the show was assembled.

The special power of the Minneapolis assemblage lay in its vast potential for aiding the unsophisticated but motivated viewer to gain insights hitherto available exclusively to the connoisseur. The expert is equipped to honor Rembrandt, for he understands the Master's technical innovations, heightened expressive powers, special use of color, unsurpassed capacity to capture an emotion and compose a scene. What the average viewer had only glimpsed in a traditional show could now become manifest; as if magically supplied with the critic's lens, he too became capable of contrasting Rembrandt with his lesser contemporaries and, more especially, with those poseurs of later periods who unsuccessfully attempted to pass for the Dutch master. And particularly when given the opportunity to examine several fakes, forgeries, and deceptions, the audience member could gain a feeling for the range and depth of Rembrandt's powers; he had the invaluable chance to survey a variety of artists, each failing (in instructive ways) to achieve a desired effect.

Derogating the fake may be unnecessarily argumentative. To be sure, when it comes to a genius of Rembrandtian proportions, almost any comparison is likely to be at the expense of the deceptive work. But prior to, and perhaps more important than, the ultimate evaluation in terms of good and bad, better and worse, is the vital capacity to *discern*, to *appreciate differences*. What renders the work effective or ineffective to the viewer is the manner in which the numerous choices and challenges confronting the artists were resolved. Viewing the finished products, we confront records of the artists' choices—the differences in the final canvases—and from these derive our final evaluation.

All judgment, all evaluation, necessarily presupposes and depends upon comparison. In most exhibitions and displays, the comparisons are implicit: the viewer must compare what he sees with what the artist might have done, given similar goals and means, but different abilities, plans, or techniques. The connoisseur is prepared for these implicit comparisons, for he has seen the absent works so many times that they have been deeply engraved on his mind's eye, but the average viewer is only rarely so equipped. At the "Fakes" show all viewers had the opportunity to be connoisseurs, for the raw materials were provided from which informed comparisons could be made and reasoned judgments achieved.

Indeed the opportunity was more than merely present: the invitation to compare was compelling. For faced with two apparent Botticellis and with the knowledge that only one is the "real thing," a virtually irresistible temptation arises to examine both closely, to peer back and forth, to focus on respective attempts to realize details, capture expressions, achieve certain hues, and, after detecting the differences, to make an informed guess about which is the "real Botticelli." Cleverly exploiting the pervasive human proclivity to enter into such a game, the Museum placed in every municipal bus a poster bearing two Mona Lisas with the enticing caption "Will the real Mona Lisa please stand up?" The stagers of the exhibit had exploited the human tendency to search for similarities and differences among objects or displays, to represent to oneself the meanings of such resemblances and disparities, and to evaluate works on the basis of such a survey. In a way, adoption of the phrase "illuminating comparisons" may yield a deceptively simplified view of this process; in fact, achievement of such comparisons is a lengthy, painstaking process, fraught with the possibility of uninstructive contrasts and misleading conclusions. By no means will any set of objects or art works lend themselves to comparisons, let alone to relevant and enlightening ones. Rather, like the physician who draws on his memory in making a rare diagnosis, a curator or instructor must search through a mental (or physical) catalogue of many hundreds of objects in order to select that pair or trio which drives home to even the most uninitiated individual the salient points of a lesson or a comparison.

Had the Minneapolis exhibition contained an endless series of originals juxtaposed to fakes, it would have been interesting and at least moderately entertaining, but not to my mind especially memorable. Again, however, the unseen hand which mounted the exhibit was guided by a basic tenet of human psychology: that there are many ways to stimulate a comparison, and that our minds are well served by a multiplicity of exploratory routes. Thus a wide array of comparisons was featured. Nearly every set of works posed a new challenge; no solution generalized automatically to the succeeding alcove; and yet there were enough possibilities for success and sufficient emerging patterns for the viewers so that, rather than despairing, they were instead stimulated to proceed on their course through the gallery.

Let me record a few of the pedagogical techniques that effectively stimulated comparisons. To begin with, one might speak of a *distance* principle: some works were directly juxtaposed to facilitate comparison; others were mounted at some remove so that one had to stroll back and forth to effect a comparison. This device brought home the lesson that the expert does not always have the original available to him; it stimulated the viewer to remember or reconstruct the original, so that he might achieve the present comparison and be better equipped for future ones. In addition to geographical distance, disparities in quality were included. Sometimes the difference between the original and fake was quite evident—so that even the least trained eye could detect it—at other times it was so subtle that supplementary aids were needed. The museum provided a magnifying glass in one such instance, and it was constantly employed by visitors.

Further cognitive exercise was insured by the inclusion of a wide variety of comparisons. The sets included, for instance, an original and a fake, an original and two or three fakes, lithographs produced in different periods, an original and a copy by a member of the artist's own school, innocently produced copies which had been provided with false signature, copies supervised by the artist himself, and a whole group of fakes collected by one individual. These assemblages revealed that the expert is continually confronted with new problems and questions, that there is no unequivocal line between fakes, forgeries, and harmless exercises. The viewer was challenged to take on the task of the expert and to learn from each of these confrontations. Every set conveyed new messages or presented old messages in slightly new ways.

Furthermore, to warn the viewer against facile conclusions, some presentations were deliberately misleading: originals without signatures; originals of poor quality; a whole set of fakes without any original. Again these unexpected twists provided special insights into the expert's dilemmas and conferred a light touch upon the exhibit as well. Finally, the show featured some unfrocked forgeries, in which the forged work is only partially removed, revealing part of the older worthless painting on top of which the forger had labored. An apparent El Greco or a Holbein which has been partially defaced served as a dramatic and jarring reminder of the manner in which forgers work.

A third distinctive feature of the exhibit was the way in which it emphasized diverse historical and stylistic features. Included were several works by a single forger (e.g., Van Meegeren) as well as attempts by different artists to imitate one artist (several fake Rembrandts). The viewer gained a feeling for the style of the forger (who often reveals his own time when sufficient examples of his work are gathered in one place) and also an appreciation for the subtlety of the original artist's style (by seeing the manifold ways in which it is possible to disfigure a Rembrandt).

Forgeries date back to ancient times, and fakes have been elicited by diverse circumstances at different epochs in history. The special problems raised by contemporary forgeries were clarified by the exhibit: we have no distance from our own era; sophisticated methods of mechanical reproduction are available; certain works (such as conceptual or pop art) seem particularly easy to duplicate, at least to our own eyes. Nonetheless, clear differences could be seen between the original and a copy of Oldenburg's *Baked Potato* (1966).

Finally, the exhibit conveyed a sense of the task an expert faces when he encounters a suspected deception. Insights were provided into the different cues available to the expert: methods of signature, size of work, age of canvas, x-ray methods, tiny details of shading, awareness of anachronistic details or colors, construction of the frame, knowledge that an artist favored certain themes and spurned others, failure to capture a certain facial expression. These methods differ greatly in their objectivity, their reliance on technology, their dependence on acquaintance with other works by the artist, but all are helpful. The exhibit

Howard
Gardner

109

also revealed that some attributions are disputed; and it illustrated how a convergence of reasons, none of which is individually decisive, can nonetheless lead to authoritative conclusions. The viewer was thus enabled to draw on multiple criteria in making his own judgments.

Though tremendously impressed with, and delighted by, the stunning exhibit, I was conscious of a number of problems that it raised. Although described as educational, it is unclear that the exhibit educated anyone. I believe that it did, and so do those at the museum, but there is no proof. It does not suffice merely to assume that displays intended to stimulate comparisons have had that effect: they may have had unintended consequences or no consequences at all. To evaluate the educational success of an exhibit, no elaborate machinery or high-power statistical techniques would be necessary: a common-sense approach and perhaps consultation with a psychologist should yield suitable and unobtrusive measures of audience learning.

Another difficulty centered around the level of audience sophistication assumed by the displayers. Though, in my view, most visitors enjoyed and profited from the exhibit, a significant number commented that it was too difficult. Some viewers failed to see differences alluded to in captions; others expressed disillusionment about the whole connoisseurial enterprise: "Well, if the experts make all these mistakes, how can I ever hope to tell?" "Who knows, perhaps half the pictures we admire are fakes." "The experts don't know any more than we do." These latter comments are particularly disconcerting. They suggest that for certain viewers the comparisons may have failed in their intended effects. True, their awe of art may have been healthily reduced, but at the bitter price of a general cynicism.

The expert's role vis-à-vis the audience is a challenging one. It does not suffice to say, "I have chosen this work: therefore you must like it." After all, the expert does not casually decide which classical vase to display: he knows and he cares about mythology, Greek methods of sculpture, the materials available to artists of two millennia ago, the clothing, religion, philosophy, mores, likes, and prejudices of individuals of that era. It is not enough simply to declare his knowledge to the viewer; such technical detail cannot be absorbed by the unprepared mind. Rather, an exhibit should be so staged that the viewer is led, subtly and entertainingly, yet authoritatively and convincingly, into the reaches of the expert's own knowledge. Only then can the nonexpert appreciate why *this* art work is worth examining today. The Minneapolis exhibit was most successful when it made the world of the expert come alive for the viewer, less successful when it simply paraded knowledge or assumed understanding.

Finally, some comments are also in order about the supplementary information sources—the labels and program guides—that adorned the exhibit. There is no question that some labeling is essential in an exhibit of this type; else how can one tell if his guesses are correct or what features to look at if he is incorrect? Without good labels, the exhibit would not work. The labels should be placed in a nonprominent spot: indeed, it might be optimal if the viewer were not allowed to scan the label until he had spent some time examining the canvas. It is too easy to conclude that you have seen what you are supposed to see after you have been told what it is and where to look for it.

In general, I encountered two difficulties with the labels in the "Fakes" show, difficulties by no means restricted to the present exhibit. First of all, there was a fair amount of technical material—recondite references to the styles of painting, characters from mythology, methods of production and detection, which were doubtless devoid of meaning to many viewers. Such references could intimidate them. Second, there was too much empty display of erudition.

An effective label is one which points to a difference which can then be seen by the viewer: "In the original the shading runs directly in the clouds; in the fake there is a gap of two millimeters"; "In the original the numeral five has been printed backwards." An ineffective label is one which is too vague or which requires specialized knowledge. I have listed some labels which I found unhelpful:

"The dullness of A vs. the vibrancy of B."

"The piece is mechanical and dull, displaying nothing of the fine concern for life and death which characterizes Aztec religion."

"The difference between the pieces is in essence, not in substance."

"While superficially Renaissance in style, the triptych is really purest nineteenth century."

"The artist expresses awe whereas the copy is merely coy."

"The forgery captures none of the subtle qualities of the original."

"Out of character in terms of the artist's true style."

"It fails to capture the artist's deeply felt religious feeling."

It might have been helpful to categorize the kinds of differences cited; at least then label-writer and viewer alike would acknowledge the differences between an objective technical reason (age of frame), an objective nontechnical reason (the shading doesn't reach to the clouds), an interpretation which is readily verified ("The Madonna in the original is looking directly into the eyes of the child"), an interpretation that does not lend itself to such verification ("The forger fails to capture the religious spirit of the original.") I do not mean to imply that the latter reason is irrelevant, only that in the present context it could have so many possible meanings that it does nothing to sharpen the viewer's appreciation.

Discussion of labels and their applicability to works of art raises the vexing question of the relationship between visual displays and linguistic instruction. The question is especially crucial in the present context, given the goal, on the one hand, of improving the viewer's perceptual skills, and the risk, on the other hand, that he fail to draw valid inferences from the comparison before him. And yet the question is extremely controversial. One school of thought is deeply suspicious of any linguistic comments about "ineffable" works of art, while another equally vociferous group considers verbal instruction the optimal means for enhancing aesthetic sensitivity.

In this dispute, the views of Rudolf Arnheim are especially instructive. As one who has devoted a lifetime to the understanding of art, and who writes eloquently on the subject, he is keenly sensitive to the advantages and the drawbacks of linguistic and nonlinguistic modes of communication. Arnheim has offered a needed corrective to the uncritical overuse, and frequent misapplication, of linguistic instruction in our educational system. Without questioning the essential communicative role of language and its appropriateness for transmitting certain subject matters, he challenges the widespread belief that language provides the optimal means for presenting the full range of information and capturing the entire gamut of thought processes. Arnheim demonstrates that thought processes rely heavily on the effective functioning of our sensory modalities and on the role of nonlinguistic symbol systems.

By theoretical conceptualization, as well as by example, Arnheim has helped to specify the appropriate role of ordinary language in explicating the arts. Often, as at certain points in the Minneapolis exhibit, the correct point will be grasped without recourse to verbal documentation; at such times linguistic elaboration is neither necessary nor desirable. At other times, however, a pictorial display may be subjected to numerous interpretations and the intended pedagogical principle, the illuminating comparison, is likely to be missed. At such times verbal labels can provide useful supplements, directing the viewer toward points worthy of his consideration, helping to explicate the significance of elements that have been but dimly discerned. The shortest distance to effective communication is not always a direct or literal line, however. Metaphors, personifications, and other figures of speech may well succeed in conveying a crucial point in an especially succinct and effective manner. Particularly in the arts, the connotative and allusive qualities of language constitute a rich resource for the sensitive teacher or writer. Certainly we must not delete words from artistic instruction; we must only deploy them with the precision and care with which a brush is wielded or a violin bowed.

A case could be made that all learning necessitates contrasts and comparisons. Where there is no change, no discrepancy, no gap, no perceived distinctions, we cannot learn. The Minneapolis exhibit overshadowed most other cultural and educational experiments because, by means of a simple yet elegant technique, the viewer was enticed into comparisons; owing to the aptness of the comparisons, significant new aesthetic insights could be gained. A simple example, or an illuminating comparison of two works, can form the beginning of a deeper understanding of a principle. But the future application of this principle requires that its underlying features be detected and formulated with some precision.

The inquiry prompted by my visit to Minneapolis suggests certain conclusions about the role of comparisons in artistic knowledge. First, the teacher or exhibitor must be clear in his own mind about what educational point is to be made and have some confidence that the point is worth making. Next, he should select a variety of examples that illustrate the point in a number of different and accessible fashions. He should consider the use of various linguistic and nonlinguistic supplements for conveying the point; and if such supplements are used, he must take care that they direct attention to the relevant details, rather than serve to obfuscate the point or to signal the brilliance of the writer. And, finally, he should engage in some modest experimentation in order to determine whether the point at issue has indeed been grasped by the intended audience. In addition to a set of guidelines like this, however, some models or exam-

Howard
Gardner

ples of effective aesthetic education are also desirable. To those in search of such models, I can point with enthusiasm to the Minneapolis exhibit and to the works of Rudolf Arnheim, in which are exemplified many of the principles touched on in this essay.

III

ARTIFACT

Various kinds of analysis of works of art are discussed in this section.

Sekler undertakes a kind of historical analysis, relating a tapestry by Le Corbusier to a whole series of other works of the artist that contain parts of the same "pictorial word." One of the elements of the very same configuration is comparable to the plan of the Carpenter Center, Le Corbusier's only building in North America, where the tapestry hangs.

In her discussion of historical influences of Gestalt psychology on the work of Paul Klee, Teuber demonstrates a direct and specific link between psychology and art. Not only are visits of Gestalt psychologists to the Dessau Bauhaus documented; actual patterns employed by Wertheimer to illustrate principles of perceptual grouping are shown to reappear on Klee's canvases. Other specific influences of the perceptual work of Gestalt psychologists are described, along with the artist's transformation of the abstract patterns of the laboratory into increasingly expressive compositions, in which form and content are no longer distinguishable.

The change in representations of the Annunciation is Zucker's subject. Since the event itself is a purely spiritual one, the artist is confronted with the problem of the representation of the invisible, whereas the scholar is concerned with the interpretation of the invisible made visible.

Hess contributes a formal analysis of a painting. By applying the golden section and other formal devices to various dimensions of a painting by Vermeer, he describes some of the factors that create the harmonious balance of shapes and colors in the complex structure of the picture.

Finally, Ashton addresses herself to those ever-present questions: Is the artist a man of his own time or does he transcend it? Is his work a social commentary or an aesthetic statement? Is the work of art the product of social change or of its own autonomous history? She concludes that there is no flat answer; the work of art is polyvalent.

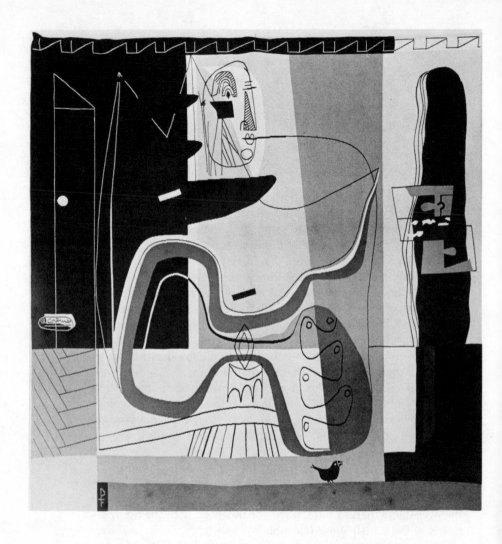

1   Le Corbusier, *La femme et le moineau*, 1957, tapestry hanging in the
main office of the Carpenter Center for the Visual Arts, Harvard
University (photo: Todd Stuart).

Eduard F. Sekler

Le Corbusier's Use of a "Pictorial Word" in His Tapestry *La Femme et le Moineau*

Ainsi des thèmes nombreux et dispersés sur l'éventail
(unique) d'un engagement plastique meublaient l'esprit
au cours de trente années. . . .

Le Corbusier, 1951

The Carpenter Center for the Visual Arts at Harvard University is Le Corbusier's only building in North America. In the Center's main administrative office hangs a large tapestry by Le Corbusier, the only work of art in the room. It is *La Femme et le Moineau*, one of an edition of six, ca. 88 × 88", done at Aubusson in 1957 (Fig. 1).[1]

The topic and the composition are closely related to a whole series of other works by Le Corbusier. These were done over a long period—from 1946 through 1964—in various techniques, and most were given the title *Icône*.[2] Among them are two drawings (Figs. 2 and 3) and a color lithograph (Fig. 4) done in 1952, thus antedating considerably three paintings on the same subject of 1955–1956, which immediately precede the tapestry. One of the drawings is in *crayon à bille* (Fig. 2); the other is in colored crayons (Fig. 3) with an inscription *"tapisserie"* in Le Corbusier's handwriting next to the date of 23 Août 52—possibly the first reference to using the *Icône* theme in a tapestry.[3]

In a painting, the imagery of the *Icône* series first occurs in *Açores 45*, a work dated 1946.[4] Here, as in the tapestry and all related works, a woman with bared breasts and large folded hands is the center of the composition; a burning candle is conspicuous in the foreground, though this feature is not included

The present study owes much to the valuable advice and help provided by my wife, Mary Patricia May Sekler, who never tired of guiding me through the intricacies of Purist painting.

119

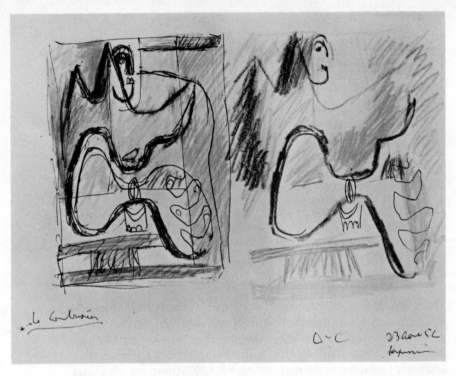

2   Le Corbusier, *Femme et bougie* (Icône), 1952, *crayon à bille* on copying paper, 27 cm x 21 cm. Courtesy ARCHIVES Fondation Le Corbusier, Paris. No. 2616. © by SPADEM Paris 1975.

in all later versions of the theme. The composition to some degree recalls *L'Ange Gardien du Foyer à la Cathédrale de Sens*, a painting of 1944,[5] but the literal derivation and meaning of the woman with burning candle become clear from a drawing that was obviously the point of departure for the whole *Icône* series: it is entitled *Pendant la Tempête sur un Cargot: Açores. 1945 (Nouvel An).*[6] The artist, on a sea voyage on New Year's Day 1945, observed a woman praying with a lit candle during a tempest; in many Catholic countries the custom survives of lighting a blessed candle during a thunderstorm in order to avert being struck by lightning. This further utilization by Le Corbusier of an impression made during a journey is typical of his method of developing one pictorial theme in several versions. It is a method he liked to describe as *recherche patiente*, and it involved not only the production of several versions of a single theme—a venerable usage, after all, in painters' studios through the centuries—but something much more drastic: a transformation

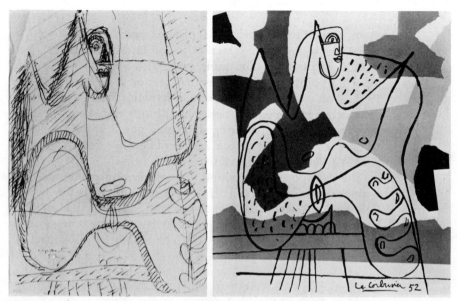

3 *(left)* Le Corbusier, *Première pensée pour sculpture*, 1952, drawing, colored crayons. Courtesy Galerie Beyeler, Basel.

4 *(right)* Le Corbusier, *Untitled*, color lithograph of *Icône* theme, dated 52, included with the series *La mer est toujours presente*, 1962.

of certain motives into something like signs or even symbols that could be used in the most varied contexts, regardless of their original derivation and meaning. This process, of obvious interest to anyone concerned with the question of possible relations between the theory of spoken and visual language, is well illustrated by one of the configurations found in *La Femme et le Moineau*, the object of our study.

Like most of Le Corbusier's pictorial work of the period, the tapestry is disciplined by a geometrical framework based on square and golden section as they are embodied in the artist's system of proportioning, the Modulor. In one of the compartments so created, to the right of the central figure, there is a configuration on yellow ground that, at first sight, is hard to understand except as an abstract constellation of angular and curving, partly transparent, forms. Upon closer study, however, one can derive every element in this portion of the tapestry from a recognizable object.

The elongated, irregularly curving form reveals its true identity when it is compared to a sketch of 1930 that depicts two found objects[7]—*objets à réaction poétique*, as Le Corbusier called

Eduard F. Sekler

121

them. One of these is a longish piece of tree bark that displays a shape and a layering so similar to the tapestry's form that no mistake is possible. The same piece also appears in modified form in a painting: in the upper left portion of *Lignes de la Main*,[8] 1930, is an elongated, otherwise enigmatic, object that forms a convincing intermediary between the original sketch and the later tapestry. Once the longish layered object in the tapestry is recognized as deriving from a piece of bark, its brown color appears particularly appropriate.

The juxtaposition of found objects eliciting poetic reactions with man-made objects such as glasses and with the human figure, all the same size (as in the painting *Sculpture et Vue*,[9] 1929) begins to occur in Le Corbusier's oeuvre at a time when Purism had come to an end and Surrealism had made its full impact felt in Paris. Found objects might even serve as points of departure for entirely new visual inventions, as he later explained: "The elements of a vision come together. The key is a stump of dead wood and a pebble. . . . By dint of being drawn and redrawn, the ox, from the pebble and from the root, became a bull."[10] It is particularly interesting that when redrawing a motif in order to transform it and to fit it into a composition, the artist would frequently employ an architectural drafting technique; he used transparent onion skin paper, which permitted working with several overlays and allowed quick copying.[11]

In the tapestry, superimposed over the middle of the piece of bark, is a configuration that in outline can be loosely described as two interlocking trapezoids, or as a trapezoid with another inverted one overlapping and on top of it. If one looks at the total image of the configuration, not just at its outline, one will notice that it implies virtual movement in addition to transparency: a counterclockwise rotation. This sense of movement derives from the two red forms inside the trapezoids, which appear to be two arms of a swastika. The dynamism of this fundamental structure is comparable to that found in the plan of the Carpenter Center itself, where two free-shape forms are arranged eccentrically on either side of a central square—again implying a twisting motion (Fig. 5). Transparency and virtual movement are, of course, found in many designs by Le Corbusier.

The left portion of our configuration looks strikingly similar to a pictorial element that twice occurs in the *Poème de l'Angle Droit* (1955), once on the color lithograph plate 93 and once as a line drawing on plate 108 (Fig. 6). Both plates belong to the sec-

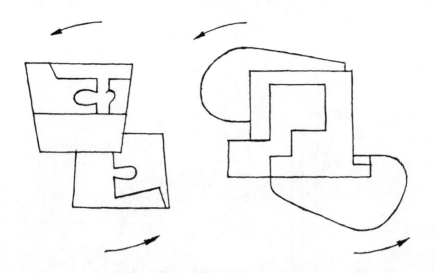

5 *(above)* Comparison of a detail from *La Femme et le moineau* with the plan of the Carpenter Center for the Visual Arts (drawing by the author).

6 *(below)* Le Corbusier, *Poème de l'angle droit*, Paris (Mourlot), 1955, Plate 108, detail.

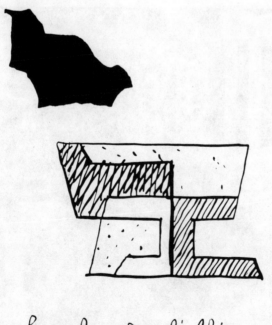

le plan de l'allégresse

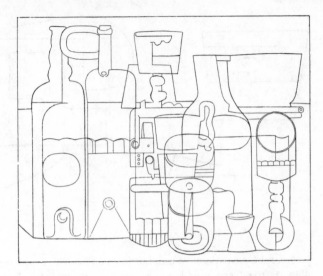

7 Jeanneret, *Still Life with Various Objects*, 1924, line cut with outlines from Ozenfant and Jeanneret, *La peinture moderne*, Paris n.d. (1925).

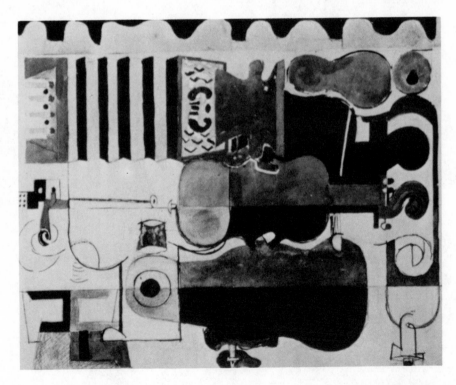

8 Jeanneret, *Lodi*, 1927, water color. Courtesy Galerie Denise René, New York.

tion C, "*Chair*," of the work, and the line drawing forms the visual conclusion to the following poetic statement: "How everything becomes strange and is transposed and projects itself high and is reflected on the plane of joy."[12]

Since the *Poème* constitutes a *summa* of convictions and images from Le Corbusier's entire artistic lifetime, pictorial motifs found in this work can often be traced back to the very beginnings of his career as a painter, when he still used his family name Jeanneret to sign his paintings. The very theme of the *Poème*, in fact, already appears in 1924 when, in *L'Esprit Nouveau*, Number 18, an article is devoted to praising the right angle. Reprinted in 1925 as part of the book *La peinture moderne* by Jeanneret and Ozenfant, the article forms part of the concluding section, where one also finds the definition and explanation of Purism, the art movement these two artists had founded. The pictorial principles of a Purist composition are illustrated on page 169 by means of a line cut (Fig. 7) that repeats the outlines of the *Still Life with Various Objects*[13] (1924), a painting that became famous because it was displayed in the *Pavillon de l'Esprit Nouveau*, 1925.

In the upper central portion of the painting and line cut (Fig. 7) there are two transparent interlocking trapezoid shapes similar enough to the configuration under discussion to qualify for consideration as its ancestor. This is quite obvious if, in addition, one looks at some intermediate links in other paintings and drawings, such as the drawing in colored crayons erroneously entitled *Accordéon et Carafe*[14] (1926) and the water color *Lodi*,[15] 1927 (Fig. 8). The forms in the upper right corner of the water color are very closely related to those in the *Poème* except that in the later lithograph of the *Poème* one portion of the outline has been omitted—the kind of elision in the service both of greater simplicity and greater ambiguity that is typical of Le Corbusier's late pictorial works.

Once one has entered the world of Purist still lifes, the identification of the two objects which in outline appear as interlocking trapezoids becomes comparatively simple. If one considers the line cut (Fig. 7) or takes a drawing such as a preparatory sketch for the *Still Life with Numerous Objects, Indépendants*, 1923,[16] and separates the two interlocking shapes, they turn out to be two stemmed glasses of the type often depicted singly in drawings and paintings of the same period. In another study for the same painting, dating from 1923 (Fig. 9), Le Corbusier even gave special prominence to a single glass. By inverting one glass

Eduard F. Sekler

125

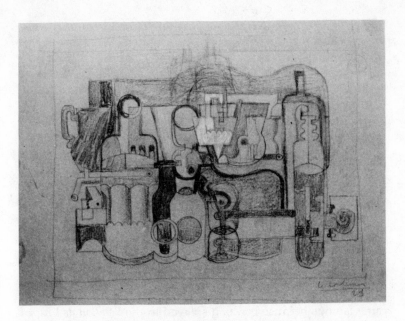

9　Le Corbusier, *Nature morte puriste avec verres et bouteilles (nombreux objets)*, 1923, black lead pencil and wax crayon on paper, 26.8 cm x 35.9 cm. Courtesy ARCHIVES Fondation Le Corbusier, Paris. No. 4685. © by SPADEM Paris 1975.

and placing it behind the other, an intriguingly ambiguous constellation of forms was created in which shared contours, transparency, reflection, and refraction (especially if one of the glasses is half filled) all helped to fulfill Purist ideals, including "the conjunction of elements with a view to creating in the painting a unique object . . . by organic arrangements."[17] Ozenfant utilized a very similar juxtaposition of two stemmed glasses in his *Still Life with a Glass of Red Wine* (1921).[18]

It is highly probable that memories of the derivation and original meaning of the "double trapezoid = interlocking glasses" motif were in the back of Le Corbusier's mind when he placed it in that portion of the *Poème de l'Angle Droit* that deals with the experiences of the "flesh" and with the "plane of joy." In obviously the same spirit, he placed the interpenetrating glasses precisely between the upturned thighs of a reclining female nude in a drawing of 1958 (Fig. 10) tellingly entitled *Ivresse;*[19] it was carried out on a portion of paper tablecloth from a restaurant at Cap Martin, his beloved Mediterranean summer resort.

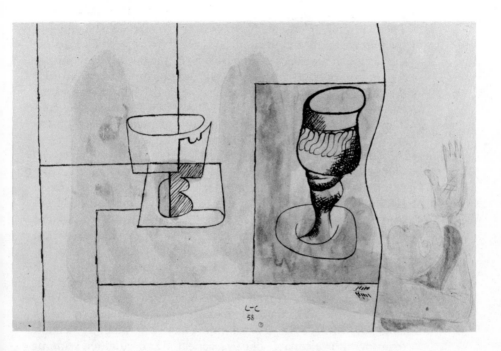

10 Le Corbusier, *Ivresse*, 1958, pen and ink with wash on paper tablecloth. Courtesy Sotheby and Co., London.

The motif of two interlocking glasses was reused and modified in many paintings and drawings and eventually became so unrecognizable that in a recent catalogue a *Still Life with Glasses and Playing Cards* (1929), which included the two glasses, was described as "machine abstraction."[20] This is understandable in view of the artist's own attitude as expressed in a statement from *L'Esprit Nouveau:*[21] "I suggest the existence of 'pictorial words' [*mots plastiques*]; the meaning of these pictorial words is not of a descriptive nature." Later this thought was elaborated in Le Corbusier's introduction to the first major publication of his pictorial oeuvre in 1938,[22] where he compared a painting to a "statement [*parole*] pronounced, heard, understood":

A statement, therefore a sentence made from words, words which carry a sense—even if hermeticism may deliberately delay its comprehension. . . . Of such word-notions two or ten may be put together. From their presence, from their diverse contiguities a relationship will be born. This relationship . . . is precisely what the artist discovers. . . .

Eduard F. Sekler

127

The method Le Corbusier implies here is one in which comparatively few significant elements are selected and modified for use in varying syntactic combinations; he applied it in his paintings where he operated with a limited number of "pictorial words" and in his architecture where "*element-types*" such as the *pilotis*, *brises-soleil*, ramps, and so on were combined in ever new contexts. His work as an architect and as a painter were always extremely closely related, as he stressed on many occasions.

More extensive studies of Le Corbusier's use of "pictorial words" and their eventual metamorphosis into architecture may contribute to a theoretical approach in the forefront of interest today: the transference to architectural analysis of methods from linguistics, structuralism, and semiology. But our present findings also pose some interesting questions of a more practical nature. If Le Corbusier's "pictorial words" were as personal in meaning as they appear to be, what are the consequences for an architectural vocabulary partly derived from them? How far can it be adopted and enlarged by others who cannot share his meanings? How far does his architecture—as opposed to the architecture of Palladio, for example—have to remain a selection of autographs incapable of being repeated and modified without being falsified? And if, for Le Corbusier and other masters of his generation, painting was indeed so important a source of forms and syntactic arrangements in space, what is the outlook for the future? In view of the direction painting is taking today, what, if any, may be its further impact on architecture?

NOTES

1. The tapestry is illustrated in Le Corbusier, *Creation is a patient search*. New York, 1960, p. 239. A color reproduction is to be found in the exhibition catalogue *Le Corbusier peintre*, Galerie Beyeler. Bâle, 1971. Professor Rudolf Arnheim was a member of the teaching faculty of the Carpenter Center from 1968 to 1974.

2. There are drawings, paintings, *papiers collés*, lithographs, and sculptures. Many of them can be found in J. Petit, *Le Corbusier lui-même*. Geneva, 1970, pp. 214–230, 249. See also Le Corbusier, *Poème de l'angle droit*, Paris, 1955, and two catalogues of the Centre Le Corbusier Heidi Weber, Zurich. *Oeuvre lithographique Le Corbusier*, n.d., Icône IV and VIII, *Papiers collés*, 1962, Nr. 9.

3. Galerie Beyeler, op. cit., Nr. 68, where the title is given as *Première Pensée pour Sculpture*.

4. J. Petit, op. cit., p. 228.

5. J. Petit, *Le Corbusier*. Lausanne, 1970, p. 72.

6. M. Jardot, *Le Corbusier dessins*. Paris, 1955, p. 65.

7. M. Jardot, op. cit., p. 33.

8. J. Petit, *Le Corbusier lui-même*, p. 220.

9. J. Petit, op. cit., p. 219.

10. *"Les éléments d'une vision se rassemblent. La clef est une souche de bois mort et un galet. . . . A force d'être dessiné et redessiné le boeuf-de-galet et de racine devint taureau."* Le Corbusier, *Poème de l'angle droit*. Paris: Mourlot, 1955, pl. 75. Translated by the author.

11. Many such sketches survive from the Purist period; others have been seen and discussed by Samir Rafi, "Le Corbusier et 'Les Femmes d'Alger'," *Revue d'Histoire et de Civilisation du Maghreb*, 1968, pp. 50 ff.

12. *"Comme tout devient étrange et se transpose se transporte haut et se réflèchit sur le plan de l'allégresse."* Translated by the author.

13. Color reproduction in M. Besset, *Who Was Le Corbusier*. Geneva, 1968, p. 61.

14. Sotheby and Co. *Fifty Works by Le Corbusier* (Sale Catalogue). London, 1969, lot 9, p. 24. The object erroneously described as accordion is a faceted glass, as can be seen by comparison with similar representations.

15. Galerie Denise René, New York. *Le Corbusier*. Exhibition Catalogue, Feb., 1972.

16. M. Jardot, op. cit., p. 13.

17. Ozenfant and Jeanneret. *La peinture moderne*. Paris, n.d. (1925), p. 168. *"La liaison des éléments en vue de créer dans le tableau un objet unique . . . par des agencements organiques."* Translated by the author.

18. M. Besset, op. cit., p. 60.

19. Sotheby and Co. *Fifty Works by Le Corbusier* (Sale Catalogue). London, 1969, Nr. 35.

20. See note 15.

21. Quoted in the excellent discussion of Le Corbusier's painting by Stanislaus von Moos. *Le Corbusier, l'architecte et son mythe*. Paris, 1971, p. 259.

22. Le Corbusier, *Oeuvre plastique, peintures et dessins, architecture*. Paris: Editions Albert Morancé, 1938. Preface.

Eduard F. Sekler

Marianne L. Teuber

Blue Night by Paul Klee

When Paul Klee (1879–1940) returned to his easel in 1937, after an illness of more than a year, he painted in a new style: his forms had become terse; his lines heavy, black, and signlike; his colored surfaces brilliant. Though the mood is often somber, here and there humorous figurative entities are lurking among abstract forms and colors. Klee's late style has presented a puzzle, but—as we shall see—perhaps no more of a puzzle than his earlier work at the Bauhaus (1921–1931), or his first abstract paintings and drawings created during World War I.

In 1935, Klee began to suffer from scleroderma, a neurological disease that makes the mucous membranes dry up, shrink, and stiffen. Ultimately, it was the cause of his death in 1940. The broad coarse lines of his late work can be attributed to the illness. But during the last three and a half years of his life, from 1937 to June 1940, Klee created an unprecedentedly large corpus of paintings and drawings: 2372 works were entered by Klee into his own oeuvre catalogue for this period. His productivity rose steadily from year to year: for 1937 Klee listed 264 works; for 1938, 489; for 1939, 1253—more than for any previous year; and for the brief period from January to April, 1940, 366 items were registered. The total figure is actually higher, for several unsigned works had not yet been entered by Klee into his catalogue. This includes his so-called last *Still Life*, which Huggler has attributed quite convincingly to late in the year 1939, instead of 1940.[1]

The Abstract Pastels

The first distinctive group of works in the new style is a series of pastels from mid- and late 1937. They are done on white cotton, burlap, and paper. The colored chalks, Grohmann states, are frequently applied to a damp ground.[2] This binds them into 131

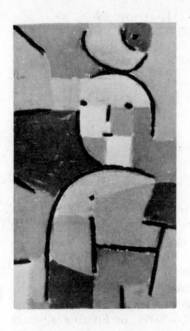

1 *Child in Red* (Kind in Rot), 1937, pastel on cotton, 13⅜ x 7⅞. Courtesy Private Collection.

more homogeneous surfaces and permits the colors to soak into the material (Figs. 1 and 3). The pastels retain, to a greater degree than the works of the following two and a half years, a purely abstract quality. Grohmann calls them mysterious—and they remain so, no matter what explanations are advanced. The dark, short, curved lines and corners indicate abbreviated forms which tend toward completion. When they become figurative, they may reveal a childlike head, as in *Figure in the Garden* or *Child in Red* (Fig. 1). These incipient shapes created by heavy, black lines are open forms. Into the openings Klee fitted terse pastel fields of strong and contrasting colors (e.g., *Figure in the Garden*). But soon he unified the picture by restricting the range of colors to immediate neighbors on the color circle. He selected one major hue for each pastel: red and its variants, several kinds of blue, yellow through orange. This beautiful restriction was entirely new to Klee's art. It can be seen in *Signs in Yellow, Child in Red, Garden in the Orient, Legend of the Nile, Stage Landscape*, all from 1937, and *Green in Green* of 1938. *Blue Night* is part of the 1937 series. It is a key work of Klee's late style.

The Picture Space of Klee's Late Paintings

Between 1937 and 1940 Klee concentrated on bringing the flat picture surface to life, a goal he had already set for himself and his students at the Bauhaus. The forms and colors stretch into the far corners of the panel (*Blue Night* or *Signs in Yellow*), as they had often done in his earlier work (e.g., *Temple of the Sect of the Green Horn*, 1917; or *At Seven over Roof Tops*, 1930). But no longer do cubelike shapes come forward and move backward from an imaginary picture plane, or float and hover over it, as in *Hovering* and *Sailing City* of 1930. The action now takes place within the two-dimensional plane, and the outlined forms are strictly two-dimensional.

Klee begins his painting by first laying out black signs and corners on a prepared ground, as can be seen in Figure 2, which shows the artist at work in his studio in Bern in 1939.[3] At other times, Klee uses untreated coarse burlap which allows the linear signs to be absorbed by the ground (*Blue Eyed Fish*, 1939, or *Death and Fire*, 1940). Then he surrounds his black outline forms, whether they are open or closed, with a new colored background.

This method of letting forms emerge from the ground had fascinated Klee before. Although the shapes themselves are different from the late sign language, *Place of Discovery* (1927) does not simply represent an archeological excavation site, known to him from his travels to Sicily and elsewhere; it is also a place where the artist discovered forms below the surface. If we look closely, we notice that the triangles, squares, diamonds are gaps in the top layer of paint. The shapes stand out, they protrude, because of the contrast effects the painter achieved through

2   Paul Klee at work, summer 1939. Photo courtesy Felix Klee, Berne.

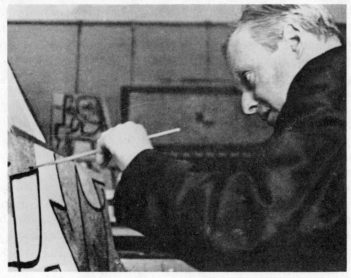

Marianne
L. Teuber

133

hatchings and shadings, a technique Klee gave up entirely in his late work.

Klee always regretted that the observer could only see the end product of his painting process, that the steps which led to it could not be retraced. For as important or perhaps more important for Klee than the finished painting was the process, the way it was made. We are not interested in form, Klee had said to his students at the Bauhaus, but in "forming."[4] Form is dead, but the aim of every painting is the growth of forms and colors on the picture plane. This concept also applies to his late style.

Origins of the Late Sign Language

Where do the signlike forms in Klee's late works come from? They have often been compared to hieroglyphs or to attempts at imitating the style of primitive cultures or the drawings of children. But at the Bauhaus Klee had explained to his students that he was not trying to become another primitive or paint in the manner of children, as certain art critics had suggested.[5] These examples of primitive or children's art, Klee said, were only another way to achieve the greatest economy of form, an attempt to penetrate "to the roots, to arrive at the beginning, at the point where forms are made."[6]

In the late thirties, in his endeavor to achieve the utmost in simplicity, Klee found a new source of inspiration—Max Wertheimer's famous essay on the "Theory of Form" (*Untersuchungen zur Lehre von der Gestalt*), published in 1923 in *Psychologische Forschung*, the journal of the Gestalt school.[7] In this essay Wertheimer tried to establish objective principles of organization which would explain why we see certain parts as belonging together and forming a unit (or Gestalt) and others not. His three major categories (or Gestalt "laws") are proximity, similarity, and good form (or good continuation). Wertheimer devised many simple patterns to demonstrate his points.[8]

If we now compare certain of Wertheimer's diagrams (Fig. 4) from his 1923 article with an almost abstract pastel by Klee, *Blue Night* of 1937 (Fig. 3), we notice that the terse black signs are shaped after Wertheimer's patterns: there are the straight horizontal lines with another line branching from the center (Fig. 4, upper left); according to Wertheimer, we see the horizontal, parts A and C, as one continuous unit, while B and C do not form a compelling configuration, though B and C are closer together than A and C. It is the form with good continuation, as

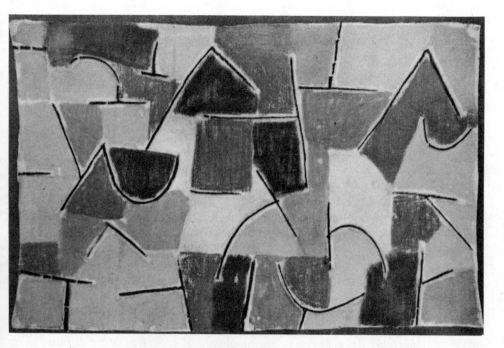

3   *Blue Night* (Blaue Nacht), 1937, pastel on cotton,
19¾ x 30. Courtesy Kunstmuseum, Basel.

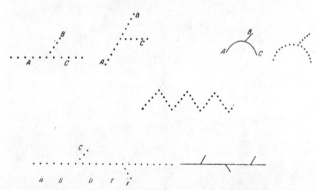

4   Max Wertheimer, *Patterns,* from *Psychologische
Forschung,* 1923. Courtesy Springer-Verlag, Heidelberg.

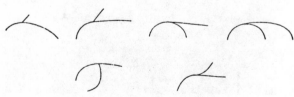

5   Max Wertheimer, *Patterns,* from *Psychologische
Forschung,* 1923. Courtesy Springer-Verlag, Heidelberg.

Wertheimer terms it, that gives the straight line its unitary quality; in this case, Wertheimer says, the principle of good continuation wins out over that of proximity. Similarly, a semicircle in Wertheimer's article (Fig. 4, upper right) and in *Blue Night* (lower right margin) follows a lawful path and is seen as a figure with good continuation, while the line branching off from the top of the curvature represents an entirely new form, as does the hooked curve departing in the opposite direction in Figure 5, second row, left. All these lines and curves, even the dotted ones (for which Wertheimer's essay was nicknamed "the dot essay"),[9] can be found in *Blue Night*. The terse pastel fields of various blues fill the space of these incipient black contour shapes that tend toward simple form.

Since Klee named his pictures only at the very end of the painting process, when all the forms and colors had joined together to produce a particular effect, it is hard to tell at what stage during the picture making the theme *Blue Night* occurred to him. The crystalline forms, extending in all directions beyond the edges, may have called to his mind passages from the *Hymns to Night*, such as " . . . but timeless and spaceless is the domin-

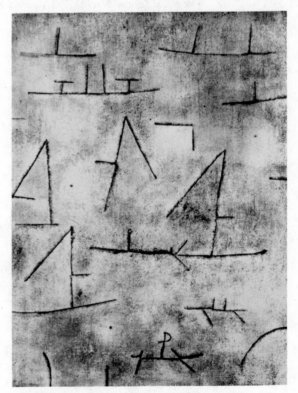

6 *Port with Sailing Ships*
(Hafen mit Segelschiffen),
1937, oil on canvas. Courtesy
Museé National d'Art
Moderne, Paris.

ion of night," by the Romantic poet Novalis, whose works Klee knew well.

The abbreviated line constructions and surfaces of Klee's late style do at times resemble script signs; at other times, primitive childlike art, as in *Figure in the Garden* or *Child in Red* (Fig. 1). They can become boats and sails as in *Port with Sailing Ships* (Fig. 6) and *Legend of the Nile* (compare Fig. 4, bottom diagrams).

However, the pastels of 1937 do not mark the first time that Klee selected patterns from Wertheimer's essay. It had captivated him before.

Experiments on Transparency at the Dessau Bauhaus

During the Dessau Bauhaus years (1925–1931) the artist employed overlapping and adjoining transparent planes from Wertheimer's and Wilhelm Fuchs' articles of 1923 for his teaching, as can be seen from Klee's Bauhaus notes (Fig. 7), where the diagrams closely resemble the Gestalt psychological patterns (Figs. 8 and 9).[10] Klee played with overlapping ambiguous abstract planes in the drawing *Rich Land* (1931, Fig. 10) and in

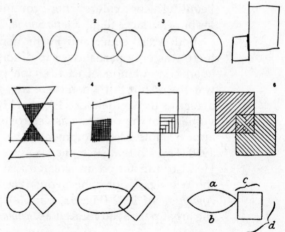

7   Paul Klee, *Overlapping and touching planes*, Bauhaus Notebooks, 1921-30, from *The Thinking Eye*, p. 117. Courtesy Schwabe and Co., Basel.

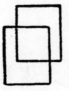

8   Max Wertheimer, *Overlapping and touching planes*, from *Psychologische Forschung*, 1923. Courtesy Springer-Verlag, Heidelberg.

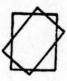

9   Wilhelm Fuchs, *Overlapping transparent planes*, from *Zeischrift für Psychologie*, 1923. Courtesy Johann Ambrosius Barth, Leipzig.

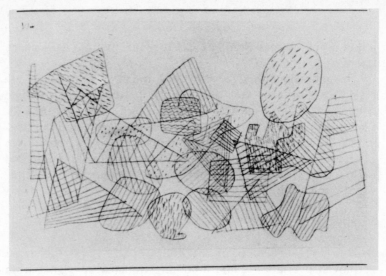

10 *Rich Land* (Üppiges Land), 1931, crayon, 20.9 x 29.5 cm. Courtesy
Collection Felix Klee, Berne.

Free but Securely Held of 1930, a painting that is clearly related to
Fuchs' experiments on transparency and Wertheimer's irregular
overlapping shapes. To this group belong also Klee's many
beautiful water colors where continuous curves result in overlapping surfaces (e.g., *Exotic Sound*, 1930).[11]

Both Wertheimer and Fuchs demonstrated that as long as
there was only partial overlap of forms (Figs. 8, 9, and 11), the
good continuation of each shape prevailed and transparency
was the result. But when there was complete overlap, as in two
diagrams of Wertheimer's Figure 11 or Klee's Figure 12, the indi-
viduality of the shapes was destroyed and transparency did not
appear. Note Klee's comment to his students at the Bauhaus in
1930 (Fig. 12) that such shapes "give up their independence."[12]
He also transferred an isolated visual motif from Wertheimer,
the two overlapping hexagons (Fig. 11) to his painting *Vegetal-
Analytical* of 1932 (Fig. 13, bottom). This was the period when
the artist portrayed himself as *Scholar* (1933).

11 Max Wertheimer, *Partially and completely overlapping planes*, from
Psychologische Forschung, 1923. Courtesy Springer-Verlag, Heidelberg.

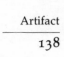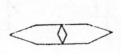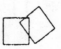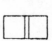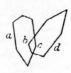

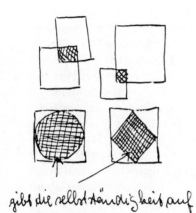

gibt die selbstständigkeit auf

12 Paul Klee, *Partially and completely overlapping planes*, from notes by Hannes Beckmann after Klee's Bauhaus course, 1930. Courtesy Professor H. Beckmann.

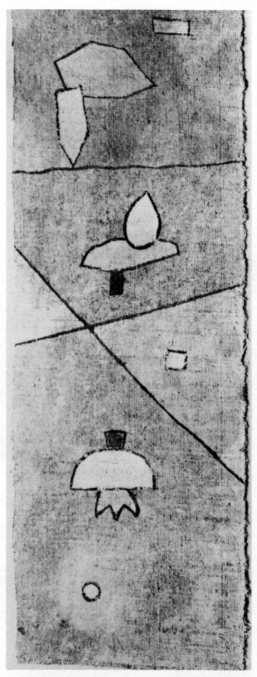

13 *Vegetal-Analytical* (Pflanzen-Analytisches), 1932, gouache on canvas, 13⅛ x 7½. Courtesy Kunstmuseum, Basel (Bequest Dr. h.c. Richard Doetsch-Benziger).

Such experiments on overlapping planes also fascinated Josef Albers, the teacher of the influential Bauhaus introductory course. He made use of these principles in his flashed glass construction *Overlapping* of 1927.[13] After he came to the United States in 1933, he developed these ideas further and passed them on to his students. In *Interaction of Color* (1963) Albers describes effects of perceptual transparency or the "illusion of transparency," as he calls it. He shows that perceptual transparency can be achieved even with opaque color papers if the overlapping shapes protrude in such a way that their "lawful" continuation can be ascertained.[14] Whereas Klee preferred the use of real transparency in his superimposed water colors and in his drawings, Albers stressed that transparency can come about with nontransparent materials, as in oil painting or in experiments with color papers. Albers created such effects of perceptual transparency in his *Bi-conjugate Series* of 1943 (oil on masonite) and *Variants on a Theme* of 1947–1948. Another demonstration of these principles can be found in *Shadows Over Yellow* (1964, Fig. 14), an oil painting by Hannes Beckmann, who was a student of Albers at the Bauhaus and again briefly in the United States.[15]

But in Klee's hands the abstract visual motifs from the psychological literature on vision do not remain abstract. He transforms them into expressive, often whimsical compositions. The functional quality of the forms themselves suggests the content, as in *Brother and Sister* of 1930 (Fig. 15). Here the transparent planes with their common areas of overlap evoke the topic. They have two sets of legs, two pairs of eyes, but *one* heart. Such visual punning is an essential feature of Klee's style.[16]

In another series from this period, the several beautiful versions of *In Angel's Keeping* (1931, Fig. 16), the overlapping planes are clearly marked as forms with good continuation by coding

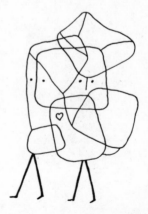

15 *Brother and Sister* (Geschwister), 1930, tracing after painting in Roland Penrose Collection, London. From Rudolf Arnheim, *Art and Visual Perception*, 1954. (Originally published by the University of California Press and Faber and Faber, Ltd; reprinted by permission.)

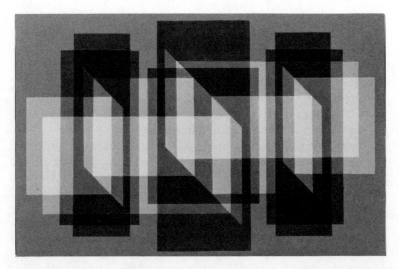

14 *(above)* Hannes Beckmann, *Shadows Over Yellow,* 1964, oil on canvas, 16 x 26. Courtesy Collection Mr. and Mrs. Harry K. Mansfield. Photo: the artist.

16 *(below) In Angel's Keeping* (In Engelshut), 1931, colored ink on paper, 16⅝ x 19⅜. Courtesy The Solomon R. Guggenheim Museum, New York.

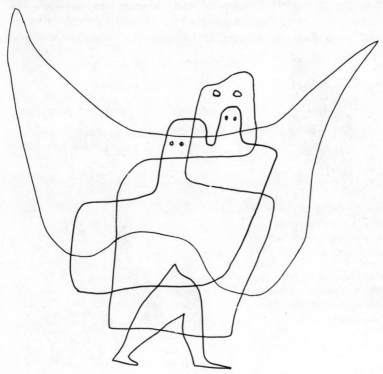

each contour in a different color. But the perceptual motifs, as nearly always in Klee's work, become transmuted by his urge to imbue them with physiognomic significance. In his lecture "On Modern Art" (1924), he had said: "Every form has its face, its physiognomy. Shapes look at us, gay or severe, tense or relaxed, suffering or smiling." The overlapping planes of *In Angel's Keeping* become a modern *Tobias and the Angel* (so often painted by Rembrandt in a completely different style).

These physiognomic transformations of his initial abstract forms and colors have obscured the fact that much of Klee's Bauhaus teaching and his picture-making is based on very personal and poetic variations of contemporary studies on vision and visual perception. His interest in these phenomena can now be traced to a period long before he joined the Bauhaus in 1921, even before he met Kandinsky in 1911.

Early Contacts with Experiments and Theories of Visual Perception

Paul Klee was twenty-five years old when he became acquainted with *The Analysis of Sensations* (1886) by the physicist and physiologist Ernst Mach.[17] The book made a deep impression on the young artist, as can be seen from his diary entries in July and August of 1905.[18] Ten years later, Mach's emphasis on the economy of form, his analyses of visual and musical patterns, and his ambiguous reversible diagrams (his so-called *book* and

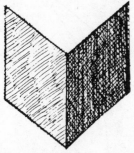

17 *(above)* Ernst Mach, *Reversible folded card (or book)*, 1886, showing the characteristic shading employed by Klee. (For credit information see Fig. 15.)

18 *(right) Untitled, Like a Vignette* (Vignettenartig), 1915, pen drawing, 19.3 x 13.7 cm. Courtesy Collection Dr. Sprengel, Hannover.

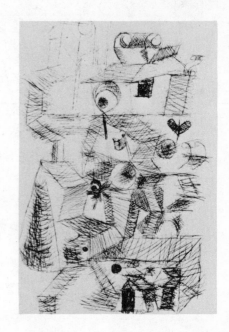

flag), contributed to Klee's first abstract compositions during World War I (Figs. 17 and 18, among many other examples). He brought these ideas with him to the Bauhaus, where his teaching during the Weimar period (1921–1924) reflected primarily the perceptual analyses of the immediate forerunners of the Gestalt school (as does the teaching of Kandinsky).[19] Diagrams and explanations in Klee's *Pedagogical Sketchbook* (1925) and Bauhaus teaching notes or in Kandinsky's *Point and Line to Plane* (1926) leave no doubt that they were fascinated by the work of F. Schumann (Wertheimer's teacher) and the theory of kinetic empathy of the Munich psychologist Theodor Lipps.

The lasting influence of pre-Gestalt theories and experiments on Klee and Kandinsky cannot be overrated. These ideas were fashionable during the period preceding their arrival at the Bauhaus—in particular the teachings of Lipps, who attracted large audiences at the University of Munich between 1894 and 1913, the very period when Kandinsky and Klee began their artistic careers in the Bavarian capital. Lipps described how, by "feeling ourselves into" forms and colors, we can experience how they expand and contract, how a movement elicits a countermovement, how "lines become carriers of motion" and emotion.[20] The many arrows in Kandinsky's diagrams (Fig. 19) and in Klee's paintings are indicators of the intrinsic movement of forms and their emotional impact; this can be seen even in a very late drawing by Klee, his striking *Burden* of 1939 (Fig. 20).[21]

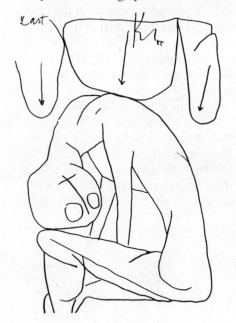

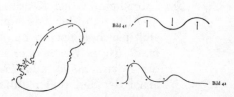

19 (*above*) Vassily Kandinsky, *Patterns*, from *Point and Line to Plane*, 1926, planned in 1914. Courtesy Benteli Verlag, Switzerland.

20 (*left*) *Burden* (Last), 1939, pencil drawing, 11½ x 8¼. Courtesy Collection Felix Klee, Berne.

But Wertheimer was not satisfied with these subjective phenomenal analyses of the forerunners of the Gestalt school. He sought
objective indices of structure when he established his "Gestalt
laws." Only during the Dessau Bauhaus years (1925–1931) and
in Düsseldorf (1931–1933) do we have evidence that Klee became interested in Wertheimer's approach and Gestalt
psychological experimentation makes itself felt in his teaching
and picture making. Among the devices which served the Gestalt psychologist in his investigation of what constitutes form (or
Gestalt), Klee employed during the Dessau period the reversal
of figure and ground (in *Departure of the Ships*, 1927), double
function of contour (in *Swinging Polyphony*, 1931), the reversible
cube (in *Santa A in B*, 1929 or *Hovering*, 1930), overlapping transparent planes. At this time Albers, too, became fascinated by
these ambiguous constellations.[22]

It was during the Dessau period that Gestalt psychologists
were invited to the Bauhaus to lecture. In 1929, Karl Duncker,
from the Psychological Institute of the University of Berlin
headed by Wolfgang Köhler, gave a lecture and demonstrations;[23] and in the winter term 1930–1931, Count Karlfried von
Dürckheim came regularly from the University of Leipzig to present an entire course on Gestalt psychology.[24] While these lectures were of great importance to the younger generation of students and faculty,[25] Klee obviously already knew what the field
had to offer and had adopted it for his own purposes. He at-
tended the lecture by Duncker, but not the course by von
Dürckheim, which Kandinsky and Albers frequently did.[26]

Although Klee was familiar with the experiments of the Gestalt psychologists in the second half of the twenties and had
made use of Wertheimer's ambiguous overlapping shapes and
other diagrams from his 1923 study, it took until 1937 before the
artist decided that a different set of experimental patterns,
namely the incipient forms (Figs. 4 and 5) were germane to his
intentions. Such long delays between the reception of intellectual and visual stimuli and their final appearance in his oeuvre
can be observed again and again throughout his artistic career.

Some Gestalt Psychological Implications of Klee's Late Style

But in 1937, when he embarked on the productive last phase of
his picture making, Wertheimer's contour diagrams (Figs. 4 and
5) and their analyses in terms of simplicity and "good continua-

tion" became an important first step in Klee's search for terse formulations, for the condensed schemata or ideograms of his late style (see *Kettledrummer*, 1940, Fig. 22 or *Als ich auf dem Esel ritt*, 1940).

While most of the pastel compositions of 1937 remain in an abstract or semiabstract state and are closely tied to Wertheimer's paradigms, Klee had already extracted figurative possibilities from these patterns in 1937, as we have seen. One should not deduce from this, however, that Klee first experimented with a motif in the abstract and then moved on to figurative transformations; these two possibilities are intermingled in his work. Thus, *Rich Land* of 1931 (Fig. 10), where he works with the interplay of abstract ambiguous planes, *follows* the figurative *Brother and Sister* of 1930 (Fig. 15). Similarly, in the 1937 series of pastels, *Blue Night* (Fig. 3), an abstract composition, is not the first of the pastels, but falls approximately in the middle of the sequence, with *Figure in the Garden, Port with Sailing Ships* (in oil), *Child in Red, Garden in the Orient, Harmonized Battle* preceding *Blue Night*, and *Signs in Yellow, Stage Landscape, Kleinode* (Jewels), *Legend of the Nile*, and *Green in Green* (1938) following it.[27]

In 1938 Klee went a step farther. He transformed the primary patterns of Wertheimer (Figs. 4 and 5), with their potential for growth and "lawful" continuation, into the luminous *Park near L[ucerne]*, Figure 21. Wertheimer's patterns become tree branches reaching upward. Light green, yellow, and red fields surround each branch indicating the area of its spreading. The bright colors and the reaching movement against a light blue ground promise spring and life, as does the sprouting plant in the center.

Klee regarded Wertheimer's patterns as *Urformen*, or primordial forms. He had spoken of such forms before at the Bauhaus;[28] similarly, his colleague and friend Kandinsky considered the triangle, square, and circle as primary shapes associated with the three primary colors, yellow, red, and blue.[29] But for Klee these forms are not static. They are only the beginning, the initial motif whence the picture develops; they will be transformed by the artist into new physiognomic entities; the process is a parable of the creation.[30] Klee's concept of growth of forms from a basic entelechy, which carries within itself the germ of its future development, is very similar to Goethe's idea of the *Urpflanze* in his *Metamorphosis of Plants*.[31] Is this one of the meanings of *Park near L*?

Klee's process of picture making usually begins with abstract

Marianne
L. Teuber

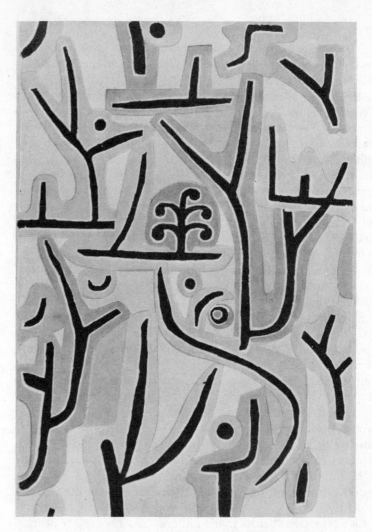

21 *Park near Lu* (Park bei Lu), 1938, oil on newspaper on
burlap, 39⅜ x 27⅝. Courtesy Paul Klee Foundation,
Museum of Fine Arts, Berne.

forms, as it does in *Park near L.* Alone or in combination, these
simple forms and colors yield a "particular constructive expression," as Klee put it in his lecture "On Modern Art,"[32] and evoke
the content of the picture; in this case memory images of trees in
a park near Lucerne.

But in the last year of his life, Klee arrived at an unusually
close coincidence of form and content in his ideograms. Stimulated by Gestalt psychological experimentation, but going far

beyond it, these terse contour compositions combine form and movement of their own accord. Arrows are no longer needed— Klee had always hoped to abolish them. The spacing of the shapes conveys rhythm as well. In *Kettledrummer* (1940, Fig. 22) we expect the vertical arm-drumstick to come down where the horizontal one has been just a moment before. Even the title, *Kettledrummer* (*Paukenspieler*) echoes the rhythm. Forms are contracted to stand for their function: the arms of the drummer become drumsticks. Form and content are one.

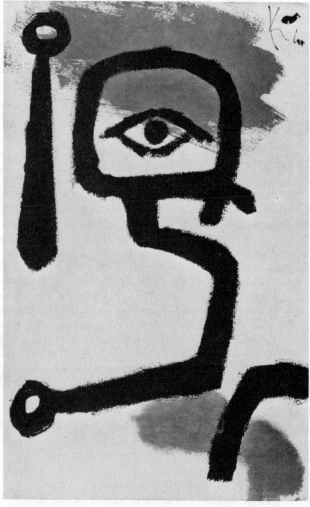

22 *Kettledrummer* (Paukenspieler), 1940, pastecolor on paper, 13½ x 8⅝. Courtesy Paul Klee Foundation, Museum of Fine Arts, Berne.

Marianne
L. Teuber

147

Conclusion

Much more could be said about Klee's contacts with experimental work on vision; but even the few instances given here suggest that Klee's teaching at the Bauhaus and his picture making can be better understood if seen as paralleling the developments in psychology and laboratory studies of visual perception (from the late nineteenth century to 1933). The rise of Gestalt psychology and its precursors left their mark on Klee. To be sure, this influence is only one facet of the artist's complex work; yet it is a side of his work that has been stressed much less than it deserves. His interest in phenomena of visual perception may not only give us a new tool for the understanding of Klee as an artist, but also cast light on seemingly obscure portions of his teaching at the Bauhaus.

NOTES

1. Max Huggler, *Paul Klee* (Frauenfeld and Stuttgart: Huber, 1969), 211–223.

2. Will Grohmann, *Paul Klee* (New York: Abrams, 1955), 336.

3. Paul Klee was left-handed. He painted and drew with his left and wrote with his right hand, as he was taught in school. His maternal grandmother, who encouraged him at the ages of three and four to draw and color, had insisted that "the child use the hand he preferred" (see Felix Klee, *Paul Klee* [Zurich: Diogenes, 1960], 35). Like Leonardo da Vinci, he wrote mirror writing with the greatest of ease. At the Bauhaus he amused his students by drawing on the blackboard with both hands simultaneously. Though Klee's paintings and drawings rarely reveal his left-handedness, his strongly hatched drawings done in the studio of his first teacher in Munich, Heinrich Knirr, in 1899, show the typical strokes of the left-hander (see Jürgen Glaesemer, *Paul Klee, Handzeichnungen I* [Kunstmuseum Bern, 1973], Figs. 201–268).

4. Paul Klee, *The Thinking Eye, Notebooks of Paul Klee I*, ed. J. Spiller, trans. R. Manheim (New York: Wittenborn, 1961), 17, 169, and elsewhere. Compare also the original German version *Das bildnerische Denken*, ed. J. Spiller (Basel and Stuttgart: Schwabe, 1956 and 1971). The 1971 third edition has the advantage of giving a clearer picture of the historical sequence of Klee's Bauhaus lectures, between 1921 and 1930; an appendix indicates whether the material comes from the first cycle of lectures of 1921–22 (BF), or from later Bauhaus folders.

5. Paul Klee, *The Thinking Eye*, 451 and elsewhere.

6. Paul Klee, "On Modern Art" (1924), in *The Thinking Eye*, 93 and elsewhere in his Bauhaus teaching notes. See also Paul Klee, *The Nature*

of *Nature, Notebooks of Paul Klee II,* ed. J. Spiller, trans. H. Norden (New York: Wittenborn, 1972), 17.

7. Max Wertheimer, "Untersuchungen zur Lehre von der Gestalt II," *Psychologische Forschung 4* (1923): 301–350.

8. See also H.-L. Teuber, "Perception," in *Handbook of Physiology: Section 1, Neurophysiology, 3,* ed. H. W. Magoun (American Physiological Society, Washington, D.C., 1961).

9. In the Psychological Institute at the University of Berlin, Wertheimer's famous essay of 1923 was nicknamed "the dot essay," since many of the patterns were composed of dots (personal communication, Rudolf Arnheim, fall 1973).

10. Paul Klee, *The Thinking Eye,* 117. Wertheimer, *Psychologische Forschung,* 1923, 325, 326. Wilhelm Fuchs, "Experimentelle Untersuchungen über das simultane Hintereinander auf derselben Sehrichtung," *Zeitschrift für Psychologie 91* (1923): 145–235. (English trans., "On Transparency," in W. Ellis, *A Source Book of Gestalt Psychology* [New York: Harcourt, Brace, 1939], 89–103).

11. *Exotic Sound,* reproduced in W. Schmalenbach, *Paul Klee* (Kunstsammlung Nordrhein-Westfalen, Düsseldorf, 1971), 69, pl. 26.

12. "...gibt die Selbstständigkeit auf," is Klee's comment. I am indebted to Professor Beckmann for giving me access to his notes of Paul Klee's Bauhaus course of 1930. A student at the Dessau Bauhaus (1929–32), Hannes Beckmann is a painter, photographer and professor of art (at Dartmouth College, Hanover, N.H.). The photograph *The Eye* is his contribution to this volume.

13. *Overlapping,* 1927, flashed glass, by Josef Albers, Collection of the Busch-Reisinger Museum, Harvard University, Cambridge, Massachusetts.

14. Josef Albers, *Interaction of Color* (New Haven and London: Yale University Press, 1963); paperback edition of text and selected plates, 1971, 24–26.

15. Note also Fabio Metelli, "The Perception of Transparency," *Scientific American 230* (April 1974): 91–98; and Metelli's article in this volume.

16. Rudolf Arnheim, *Art and Visual Perception* (Berkeley and Los Angeles: University of California Press, 1954); paperback editions since 1965. See also Marcel Franciscono, "Paul Klee's Italian Journey and the Classical Tradition," *Pantheon 32* (Jan.-March, 1974): 54–64. Franciscono calls attention to early evidence of "visual punning" in Klee's satirical etchings of 1904–1905. The absurd verses and puns of the Munich poet Christian Morgenstern, whose *Gallows Songs* (1905) Klee admired, are the closest parallel to the artist's punning with forms.

17. Marianne L. Teuber, "New Aspects of Paul Klee's Bauhaus Style," introduction to *Paul Klee: The Bauhaus Years, 1921–1931* (Des Moines, Iowa: Art Center, 1973); also, M. L. Teuber, "Paul Klee: Abstract Art and Visual Perception," paper and abstract, *61st Annual Meeting of the College Art Association of America,* New York, January 1973.

Marianne
L. Teuber

18. Paul Klee, *The Diaries of Paul Klee, 1898–1918,* ed. Felix Klee, trans. P. B. Schneider, R. Y. Zachary, and M. Knight (Berkeley and Los Angeles: University of California Press, 1964), entries 664–700 (for 1905). German edition, *Tagebücher von Paul Klee, 1898–1918,* ed. Felix Klee (Cologne: DuMont Schauberg, 1957).

19. Klee joined the Bauhaus at Weimar in January 1921, and Kandinsky in the Summer of 1922.

20. Theodor Lipps, *Raumaesthetik und geometrisch-optische Täuschungen* (Leipzig: Barth, 1897); *Aesthetik, 1* and *2* (Hamburg and Leipzig: Voss, 1903 and 1906).

21. See also Rudolf Arnheim, "The Gestalt Theory of Expression," *Psychological Review 56* (1949): 156–171. (Reprinted in R. Arnheim, *Toward a Psychology of Art: Collected Essays* [Berkeley and Los Angeles: University of California Press, 1966], paperback 1972).

22. Marianne L. Teuber, "Perceptual Art," paper and abstract, *59th Annual Meeting of the College Art Association of America,* Chicago, January 1971.

23. Hannes Meyer, "Open Letter to Lord Mayor Hesse of Dessau,"*Das Tagebuch,* Berlin, *11* (13), August 16, 1930 (reprinted in H. M. Wingler, *The Bauhaus,* [Cambridge, Mass.: M.I.T. Press, 1969], 163–165). "Dr. Dunker (sic), Berlin" is listed among the prominent lecturers, such as R. Carnap, O. Neurath, H. Prinzhorn, H. Richter, and others, invited by Hannes Meyer, director of the Bauhaus from 1928 to 1930. Most likely, the original invitation from the Bauhaus had been addressed to Wolfgang Köhler. But in the Summer and Fall of 1929 Köhler was in the United States, attending the International Congress of Psychology at Yale University and giving guest lectures in various parts of the country (conversations with Mrs. Wolfgang Köhler, 1970–1973).

24. Hannes Meyer, "Open Letter," in Wingler, *The Bauhaus,* 164: "For the winter 1930/31 an elementary course in Gestalt psychology was decided upon, in conjunction with Professor Felix Krueger, Leipzig, and his circle." See also *Notes on the Psychology Lectures* given by Dr. Karlfried von Dürckheim, 1930–31, in Wingler, *The Bauhaus,* 159–160. The notes (in the Bauhaus Archive of the Busch-Reisinger Museum, Harvard University, Cambridge, Mass.) were kept by Howard Dearstyne, then an architecture student at the Bauhaus, who studied under Ludwig Mies van der Rohe. From Dearstyne's notes it appears that von Dürckheim gave a rather complete survey of the then available Gestalt psychological literature from the point of view of the Leipzig School.

25. Hannes Beckmann, "Formative Years," in *Bauhaus and Bauhaus People,* ed. E. Neumann (New York: Van Nostrand Reinhold, 1970), 195–199. Beckmann gives a lively description of Albers' teaching at the Bauhaus and notes the impact made by von Dürckheim's lectures on Gestalt psychology.

26. Personal letter, Dr. K. von Dürckheim, spring 1971.

27. I am indebted to Dr. Jürgen Glaesemer, Klee Foundation,

Berne, for a listing of the 1937 pastels from Paul Klee's Oeuvre Catalogue.

28. Paul Klee, "On Modern Art," in *The Thinking Eye*, 93; *The Nature of Nature*, 17.

29. Vasily Kandinsky, *Punkt und Linie zu Fläche* (Point and Line to Plane), Bauhaus Book, 1926; new 5th edition with introduction by Max Bill, Berne: Benteli, 1964, 79.

30. Paul Klee, "Schöpferische Konfession," in *Tribüne der Kunst and Zeit*, ed. Kasimir Edschmid (Berlin, 1920); reprinted as "Creative Credo" in *The Thinking Eye*, 79, and elsewhere in his Bauhaus teaching notes.

31. Johann Wolfgang von Goethe, *Die Metamorphose der Pflanzen*, 1790. Hans Driesch, who came from the nearby University of Leipzig to lecture at the Weimar Bauhaus, propounded similar ideas.

32. Paul Klee, "On Modern Art," in *The Thinking Eye*, 91.

ACKNOWLEDGMENTS

It is a pleasure to thank the museum directors and curators who gave me access to various Klee collections. In particular, I am indebted to Dr. Hugo Wagner, director of the Art Museum, Berne, and to Dr. Katalin von Walterskirchen and Dr. Jürgen Glaesemer, curators of the Paul Klee Foundation, whose assistance was indispensable; to Dr. Franz Meyer, director, and Dr. Z. Felix, curator, Art Museum, Basle; to Professor Werner Schmalenbach, director, Collection Nordrhein-Westfalen, Düsseldorf; to James T. Demetrion, director, Art Center, Des Moines, Iowa; to David Farmer and Hedy B. Landman, curators, Busch-Reisinger Museum, Harvard University, Cambridge, Mass. My special thanks go to Mr. Felix Klee who guided me through his magnificent collection of paintings in Berne.

I should also like to express my appreciation to Oxford University for granting me reader's privileges in the Oxford libraries during the academic year 1971–72, when my husband was the Eastman professor (of psychology) and when I had the time and opportunity to start work on this project and related topics.

Finally, I am most grateful for helpful information provided, either in conversation or by way of correspondence, by Anni and Josef Albers, Rudolf Arnheim, Elsa and Hannes Beckmann, Lois Swirnoff Charney, James T. Demetrion, K. von Dürckheim, Jürgen Glaesemer, E. H. Gombrich, Mrs. Walter Gropius, Leo Hurvich and Dorothea Jameson, Gyorgy Kepes, Felix Klee, Andreas Köhler, Mrs. Wolfgang Köhler, K. von Walterskirchen, Mrs. Heinz Werner, and particularly, my husband, Hans-Lukas Teuber.

Marianne L. Teuber

Wolfgang M. Zucker

The Representation of the Invisible: Reflections on Christian Iconology

Someone shows me a stack of snapshots. I look at them and ask: "Who is this?" or "What is that?" The photographer is not astonished by my question; his answers come easily: "This is a Sicilian farmer praying before the shrine of a saint"; "This is the house where my mother was born." The photos may be clear or unclear, attractive or uninteresting, original or conventional; in any case they represent something, and what they represent is their content. The persons or objects depicted were apparently meaningful for the photographer: he may have wanted to show the piety of the poor in Sicily or the simplicity of the life of his grandparents. If he is a good photographer, his pictures will convey the meaning to me also, but rightly or wrongly, their "meaning" is located in the objects represented and not in the way they are represented. This is true even when, for whatever purpose, the photographer deliberately falsifies reality: a photo of a prison cell can be used to give the impression that the prisoners are mistreated or, on the contrary, that they are treated too leniently. The impression will depend on the selection of the objects represented, but the objects must have been there. They are "objective."

A very different concept of "content" and "meaning" is presupposed in the attitude of modern artists and aestheticians who regard the naïve questions "What is it?" "What does it mean?" as pedestrian and inapplicable to art. Sometimes this rejection is expressed by the forbidding statement: "A work of art does not mean—it is."

The purpose of this paper is not to argue for or against this claim. Rather it deals with art objects that were created with the intention of making religious contents visible and conveying to viewers the meaning of the Christian faith. The art of identifying the contents and understanding their meaning is the task of what has traditionally been called "iconography," but should, 153 more accurately, be called "iconology." (The craftsman who creates icons—visual images of sacred persons, objects, or events—is an iconographer; the scholar who interprets the content and meaning of the icons is an iconologist.)[1] Iconology is a special field of hermeneutics, the art of interpretation,[2] and as such faces the same difficulties. All hermeneutical work deals with "meaning" on two different levels: on the first, what is given, a text or an image of the past, must be understood with regard to what it says directly; the text must be translated from an unfamiliar language into a familiar one, the visually represented objects must be recognized. The second level of understanding is concerned with the meaning of the philosophical, religious, moral, or even aesthetic message that text and image had for a public not in need of translation. The two levels are mutually interdependent: obviously no text can be interpreted if its language is not known, but neither can a language be adequately translated unless the meaning of what is said in it is understood. Thus all hermeneutical work is always in a sense circular. No text, no image presents it own explanation, yet all explanations must be based on what is given as the material to be explained.

Until recent times the term "hermeneutics" was used only by theologians explaining the proper meaning of the sacred texts. Since the early Christian centuries, they were quite aware of the "hermeneutical circle." What the texts said could be understood only if the interpreter read it "with the eyes of faith," but faith itself was founded in and sustained by what the texts said. What was said pointed to what was not said; what was not said was needed to understand what was said. In the early history of Christian hermeneutics the dilemma manifested itself in the controversies between the hermeneutical schools of Antioch and Edessa, on the one side, and the school of Alexandria, on the other. The former, biblical philologists, emphasized the lexigraphical, grammatical, and historical side of the problem; the latter group consisted of allegorists and symbolists who diligently and with much fantasy looked for mutual relationships between different passages concealed in metaphors and sometimes in single words, by this method constructing a complicated network of meanings and explanations that supported each other.

This allegorism, this search for significant meaning behind the given text, did not begin with Christianity, nor was it confined to it. For about two centuries before Christ, scholars in

Alexandria had been engaged in what they called the "Therapy of the Myths," an attempt to interpret the incredible mythological stories of the epic poets as fanciful allegories of philosophical, moral, astronomical, or meteorological theories. This movement took a new turn with the work of Philo of Alexandria (ca. 40 B.C.–40 A.D.).[3] Philo tried to show that the sacred Hebrew Scriptures corresponded in all details to the theories of Plato, but in contrast to the Greek Therapists, he insisted at the same time on the literal truth of the biblical texts. Thus he established a hermeneutical theory of a twofold message of the Scriptures. In this he was followed by the Alexandrian School of Christian exegesis;[4] yet the doctrine has presented considerable difficulties from the time of Clement of Alexandria (ca. 150–215 A.D.) up to the controversies raised by Bultmann and his followers in our own time. An outright denial of the historical factuality of at least some core of the biblical texts puts the theologian outside of the Judaeo-Christian tradition; on the other hand, the texts themselves point to a meaning beyond the literal one. Origen (ca. 185–254), the most audacious follower of Clement, tried to resolve the difficulty by claiming that the biblical texts could be understood both "in the flesh" (literally) and "in the spirit" (allegorically), but there is no doubt that he considered the latter way as the more "faithful." This preference, which brought him into dangerous proximity to the heresy of gnosticism, made him deeply suspect to the more literal-minded theologians like Theodore of Mopsuestia (ca. 350–420), Diodorus of Tarsus (d. ca. 390), and St. Chrysostome (ca. 347–407), who rejected Alexandrian allegorism. In spite of his strong influence on Ambrose, Augustine, and even Thomas Aquinas, he was never granted the honorific epithet of "Doctor of the Church."[5]

This excursion into biblical hermeneutics is necessary to understand the fundamental problems faced both by Christian iconography and iconology. By its very definition, the visual presentation of sacred subjects must meet a double demand. It must translate the contents of a sacred text into a concrete image, and, simultaneously, let the image indicate a deeper significance which always transcends the visible object. Superficially, the inherent difficulty of the task seems to parallel that presented by verbal representation of the same subject matter, but the differences are considerable. First of all, language is itself already metaphorical. Words are not icons of their referents but symbolic signs of their meanings; unless they are name tags for

Wolfgang
M. Zucker

individual designata, they apply to a multitude of different individual objects. They easily vacillate between the general and the specific, the abstract and the concrete, the overt and the hidden. Language can speak of the invisible, whereas an image is always restricted to visible form. Secondly, a sacred text is never explicit in its details; its very brevity and vagueness often signal the presence of something that is not said and, perhaps, cannot be said. Finally, the verbal utterance and its hermeneutical interpretation are two separate processes: the interpreter says something that the author had not said because he could not say it. By contrast, the visual artist may use his material metaphorically, but the objects—a woman with a child, a tree, a wild animal—are not themselves metaphors; they are things of this world, in their appearance indistinguishable from other nonsacred things. When the artist chooses among the visual objects of the world and uses certain ones as metaphors for the representation of a religious message, he is already practicing hermeneutics. As a craftsman he is able to make images of concrete things; as the artificer of religious images, he is an interpreter.

There exists yet another factor essential to Christian art. The Christian artist does not merely illustrate the words of a given text; he simultaneously tries to make visible the meaning of the concrete persons and things that appear in his illustrations. In this sense the concept of the nature of Christian art is the exact opposite of the modern fashionable aesthetic theory referred to above. Whereas the contemporary artist and his interpreter claim that visual images "do not mean, but are," the Christian artist and his theological client believe that the things of the world not merely are, but mean. In this understanding of reality, all objects existing in the world, and therefore representable by images, are themselves signs and symbols both of other objects and of the meaningful order of the totality of the world. Every part of reality points beyond itself to other parts which are themselves symbols which point to other symbols, and so on until the totality of all things forms an intricate fabric of relationships and connections.[6]

It was more than a thousand years later that the view of the world as a network of "significationes allegoricae," as Augustine called the mutual references and connections of all things, was expressed as a philosophical theory by thinkers of the Renaissance. For Paracelsus the whole of nature was a "scriptura," a cryptic text that the philosophical scientist must learn to decipher. He wrote his books at a time when this view had reached the height of its influence and was soon to be replaced by modern explanatory science for which natural objects do not "mean," but simply "are."

Christian theologians and the artists whom they commissioned were deeply steeped in this universal allegorism. They had adopted it from both their Jewish and pagan Hellenistic teachers. In their attempts to defend the message of the Gospels against Jewish and Gentile philosophers, they tried to prove that the sacred events proclaimed as the Good News had been "prefigured" in the events of the Old Testament. Thus the sacrifice of Isaac was paralleled by the Crucifixion, Sarah by the Virgin Mary, Jonah in the belly of the whale by Christ's descent into hell, the Passage through the Red Sea by the Baptism of Jesus, etc. As the first "New Man," Christ is of the same "typos" as Adam, the first "Old Man"; Aaron is of the same type as Peter, while Eve and Mary are "antitypes."[7]

Sometimes the symbolic cross-connections seem to be farfetched and artificial, especially when they are based on intermediate links of similarities. To modern readers this hermeneutical method will appear as a kind of game with concepts and images that combine and separate in infinite variations and allow the interpreter to find references to anything in everything. (The allegoristic games played by some contemporary psychoanalysts are of the same nature, surprising, at times shocking, vaguely elucidating, and rarely quite convincing.)

Allegorical parallels were not restricted to scriptural texts. On the one hand, popular traditions expanded and extended the archaic brevity of the biblical stories with colorful details and embellishments; on the other hand, motifs from the mythologies of the ancient and Hellenistic cultures entered into the speculations of Christian thinkers.[8]

Like the Jewish Hagadah texts, these excursions into nonbiblical sources could not claim doctrinal authority but, in general, the Church was rather tolerant of them except when they were used to promote ideas condemned as heretical. Some of the traditions, though not supported by any biblical passage, became so popular and were accepted over so wide a geographical area that the difference between apocrypha and canon became obscure. Examples that still survive are the "three kings" of the Christmas story (the Gospels speak only of an unspecified number of wise men), or St. Anna, the mother of the Virgin (the

Gospels do not mention her at all). The additional material again lent itself to allegorical interpretation and cross-connections with other symbols and significations.

Needless to say, besides folk tales and legends of various origin, popular nonreligious rituals, medical practices, and magical folk customs also mixed easily with religious concepts. The erotic poetry of the Song of Solomon had already been incorporated by the Jews into the canon of religious readings (kethubim) and had been interpreted by Rabbi Akiba as a metaphor for God's love for His Chosen People. Christian exegetes from Hippolytus and Origen to Bonaventura took over this allegory enthusiastically and transferred it to the mystical marriage of Christ to his bride, the Church. The sensual imagery of this book supplied additional visual motifs for iconographers and further allegorical material for iconologists.

The development of patristic allegorism and typology and the acceptance of legendary material into theological writings, preaching, and liturgy made the work of the religious artist both more complex and visually more concrete. He now had "something to work with." Though the artists themselves probably discovered or invented the symbolic allusions only in exceptional cases, they had at their disposal the writings of the theologians and the visual suggestions made by other painters and sculptors. As a consequence, certain iconographic conventions developed, sometimes restricted to specific regions, sometimes imitated and expanded over considerable distances.

At first the didactic task of presenting biblical parallels (types, prefigurations) was met by the juxtaposition of related biblical scenes on the same page of an illuminated bible or prayer book, on the same wall of a church, or in the sculptural program of a cathedral portal. This method is followed strictly in the so-called "Biblia Pauperum,"[9] a type of book containing illustrations of biblical stories in which a scene from the New Testament is always flanked by two typologically "corresponding" scenes from the Old Testament.

The title given to these books indicates a somehow condescending attitude to religious art. At first handwritten, later printed, they were meant for the "poor in spirit," i.e., for those who were unable to read, especially for uneducated preachers as a "visual aid" in composing their sermons. Visual art was considered, in the high and late Middle Ages, as an inferior substitute for the subtle verbal game of symbols. It was different with those paintings that skillfully interwove a great number of allegorical allusions in one and the same pictorial space. They could be fully understood only by an elite group of sophisticated scholars acquainted with the literary tools of exegesis, or at least with encyclopedic works like the *Speculum Majus* of Vincent of Beauvais (1190–1264) or the *Legenda Aurea* of Jacobus de Voragine (1228–1298)[10] that summed up the whole legendary and symbolic material of the past.

Symbolic meanings are never private; they presuppose a community that understands what is meant. (Only the subjectivism of nineteenth and twentieth-century aesthetics condones and praises the "originality" of individual artists and grants them the right to a personal symbolism.) The community addressed by the artists of the high and late Middle Ages was then comparatively small. Nevertheless, their works were publicly displayed and admired. (Probably it is no different in the case of the masses of visitors to our contemporary museums. Without the title plates under the exhibits of religious art works, they would hardly know what sacred scene or person is represented, to say nothing of the symbolic meaning once intended. They may be amused when a guide informs them that the painters of Siena avoided the traditional lily in their representations of the Holy Virgin because it was the flower of the city of Florence, Siena's arch competitor—but they would still be ignorant about the relationship of the lily to the Virgin Mary.)

Yet it seems that religious symbols in a religious environment can be meaningful even when they are not understood. For the churchgoer the wall paintings and altarpieces were not works of art but objects of worship. As the mysteries of faith need not be resolved in order to be accepted, the puzzles and charades of the holy images did not require an explanation in order to be effective. The images and symbols repeated themselves from one locality to another, from altarpiece to altarpiece. The public knew the visual vocabulary without being aware of all its meanings. It seems that in some cases the artists used it like a set of traditional formulas, even when its original significance had already been forgotten. Thus at times strange combinations of very different concretizations and localizations resulted, and while the learned iconologist could give an explanation of every single detail, the iconographer, the artist, working both from models he had seen and according to the special wishes of his clients, used his skill merely to bring them all together in the one visual space of his painting. There were manuals for religious artists that informed them of the correct ways of representing

Wolfgang
M. Zucker

159

holy themes. Such handbooks may have had greater authority in the Eastern Church—where the workshops of painters of icons were more closely tied to the religious institutions—than in the west. In the west too, however, the authority of the Church sometimes interfered with the work of the artist by prohibiting the use of certain symbolic conventions. The Council of Trent (1545–1563) was quite explicit in its decrees prohibiting such iconographic subjects as the Virgin with breasts exposed suckling the Christ Child, the Giant Christopher carrying the Christ Child on his shoulders, and the Lady of Compassion spreading her coat over a large group of minute petitioners.[11]

The analysis thus resembles the work of a geologist. The iconologist must distinguish between the different layers of artistic, legendary, symbolic, and doctrinal traditions and reconstruct the development of the representation of a specific religious subject. This history is not straightforward; motifs appear and are abandoned, to re-emerge suddenly at a much later time, when they are no longer understood in their original significance and have changed into new meanings or are preserved simply as archaic visual memories. The fate of symbols is not different from that of words. Both carry their historical past with them like a hidden dimension which makes its reality felt when their use as conventional formulas itself becomes the subject of meditation.

In the remainder of this paper an attempt will be made to illustrate the different levels of signification discussed above with the example of the representations of the Annunciation.[12] The topic is especially suitable for analysis because the sacred event itself, as told in the New Testament (Luke 1: 26–38), is of an entirely spiritual nature. No other action is described than the exchange of words between the Archangel Gabriel and Mary. On the angelic salutation and the answering words of the Virgin several most significant doctrines of Catholic orthodoxy are based, but the biblical report is completely abstract.

The earliest visualizations of the Annunciation in the Roman catacombs only show a woman listening to a man whose raised hand indicates that he is speaking to her. There is no background; the visual space is left as undefined as it is in the biblical words. Only the fact that the painting (Catacomb of Priscilla, fourth century) appears among other more picturesque scenes from the New Testament allows us to identify the two figures as Gabriel and Mary.

A new level of visualization was reached under the influence of an apocryphal expansion of the biblical text, the so-called Protoevangelium of James.[13] Written at the end of the second century, it embellishes the scene with many details that lend themselves to pictorial representation. The book begins with the story of the Immaculate Conception of the Virgin Mary, continues with her growing up in the Temple and her betrothal to Joseph, and ends with the birth of Jesus. According to the unknown author, the Annunciation takes place when Mary, as a trust of the High Priest, is charged with weaving the purple part of the veil that separates the Holy of Holies from the outer room of the Temple. Going with a pitcher to a spring or well in the garden to fetch water, she hears the voice of an invisible angel; in fear she retreats into the Temple, where the now visible Archangel announces to her her election in the exact words of the Gospel according to Luke. Her answer, first of fear, then of obedience and acceptance, likewise follows the biblical text. The Protoevangelium soon became very popular, especially in the east where it underwent further legendary enlargements,[14] but it was banned in the west by decree of Pope Gelasius (d. 395), after Jerome had rejected it because of the appalling details of the testing of Mary's virginity after the birth of Jesus. In spite of this interdiction, artists continued to avail themselves freely of the legendary material. Its content, without the offensive passages, was taken over in numerous Lives of the Virgin and was incorporated in the *Legenda Aurea* which remained the authoritative source for all iconographic and hagiographic art through the later Middle Ages and the Renaissance. Finally, in 1570, the Flemish theologian Molanus (Meulen), summing up the decisions of the Council of Trent, denounced the popular book as heretical.[15] In the west the scene at the spring in the garden was rarely represented. An example is an ivory diptych of the fifth century; it shows a corporeal angel behind the Virgin with the water pitcher, although the text says that he was invisible. Shortly afterwards the illustration seems to have disappeared completely, but the ambiguity of the locality of the sacred event was preserved in later representations. It became a convention to fuse the two annunciations by placing the angel and the Virgin Mary under separate arches of a loggia or pergola, thus combining the outside of the garden and the inside of the Temple.

At the same time, however, the concreteness of the places undergoes a symbolic transformation. Both the garden with the water well and the Temple are understood not merely as envi-

Wolfgang
M. Zucker

ronment, but as visualizations of theological allegories supporting the increasing liturgical significance of the Blessed Virgin. The Temple is identified with the Holy Church; thus, especially in France and the Netherlands, the scene of the Annunciation is moved to the inside of a cathedral or chapel. The reason is that in the Mariology of Ambrose and his symbolistic followers, the Mother of Christ was herself identified with the Church.[16] It is in the Church that Christ is conceived and born in the heart of the believer. The Church is the womb of Christianity.

The garden has another symbolic dimension: it is the hortus conclusus, the locked garden with the sealed fountain, the well of living water, of which the Song of Solomon (4:12–5:1) sings, interpreted as the symbol of chastity and virginity. Though the Annunciation itself no longer takes place in the garden, the abandoned scenery is still indicated by flowers and/or a well in paintings up to the sixteenth century.[17] In far more general use is a vessel with or without flowers placed between the angel and Mary. It is usually referred to as a "vase," a mere decorative object, though when the flowers are white lilies, iconologists see in them a symbol of purity. But quite often the vessel has a spout; thus it is a pitcher rather than a vase, a visual memory of the old motif of Mary receiving the call when she goes to fetch water.[18]

The water symbolism of the Church Fathers is so rich that no artist representing the Annunciation could have been oblivious of the significance of the water vessel. In patristic typology the Flood and the Passage through the Red Sea were prefigurations of the baptism of Jesus and therefore of every Christian. The connection to the "Rivers of Living Water" flowing out of the body of Christ[19] was established early. What in the story of Mary's youth was an object of profane use became in the iconographic translation the symbol of a sacred mystery, the spiritual life, received by the Christian in baptism and constantly renewed through the sacraments and the sermons of the Church. The outsides of the wings of the Ghent Altarpiece show the Angel of the Annunciation and the Virgin in a large but low room with arched windows overlooking a medieval city. But the space between the wings preserves the memory of earlier iconographic modes: on the left, two arches of a pergola, on the right, a holy water font hanging in a tabernacle.

While the allegoristic connections and cross-references develop to greater and greater complexity, the tendency toward realistic concreteness also increases. The question of what the Virgin Mary was doing when the angel appeared to her is answered in various mutually exclusive ways. After the scene at the spring or well had disappeared in the west, three solutions seem to have been popular. The oldest, still following the story of the Protoevangelium, presents Mary spinning the purple thread for the veil of the Temple. Thus the Virgin holds in her hand either a spindle from which she draws out a thread (e.g., Mosaic in S. Maria Maggiore, Rome, 440 A.D.) or a skein (West Portal, Notre Dame, Paris). In the "Byzantine Guide to Painting" which A.N. Didron published from a late manuscript found in a monastery on Mt. Athos, the instruction to the painter reads: "The Holy Virgin standing before a seat, her head a little bent. In her left hand she holds a spindle with silk rolled on it; her right hand is stretched out open towards the Archangel. . . ."[20]

The spindle motif becomes rare after the fifth century. Instead the Virgin is shown reading when the Archangel Gabriel appears to her. In some representations the words of the book can be seen clearly. They are taken from Isaiah 7:14: "Ecce, virgo concipiet in utero et pariet filium et vocabitur nomen eius Emmanuel." While writers at the end of the Carolingian period already reported that Mary, at the moment of the Annunciation, was reading the Bible, the *Meditationes* of the Pseudo Bonaventura (end of the thirteenth century) identified the precise passage as the prophecy of Isaiah.

The book remained an attribute in most representations of the Annunciation even when, in later paintings, the event was placed at the entrance door of a church as, for example, in the Annunciation of the Friedsam Collection of the Metropolitan Museum in New York, dated ca. 1425.[21]

While the change of location from the garden to the loggia and to the inside of a church was based on the extensions of the Protoevangelium, the placing of the Annunciation in the bedroom of the Virgin was, for two reasons, independent of the ancient legendary material. One was the spreading recognition of the Holy House of Our Lady at Loreto. According to a tradition beginning in the fourteenth century, the house in Nazareth where the Annunciation had taken place was miraculously carried by angels, via Dalmatia, to the Italian town of Loreto in 1291. The simple room around which a pilgrimage church was built became the physically real model for a new mode of representation, in which the interior of a small house is skillfully integrated into the architecture of a Gothic church.[22] The other decisive influence on the new iconography, not only of the Annunciation but of all religious subjects, was the "world piety" of the Franciscan movement in the fourteenth and fifteenth centuries—a loving acceptance of the humble profane world and all its living and inanimate objects. The artists began to fill the room in which the Virgin receives the messenger of God with the objects of everyday bourgeois life—a bed with one of the curtains rolled up, a prie-dieu, a candlestick, a water bowl with a slightly rumpled towel beside it. All the objects, of course, also have an allegorical and symbolic significance, but the artists, especially in northern France and the Netherlands, seem to have delighted in the "thingness" of the real objects depicted. The hierarchic, ecclesiastic, courtly style of earlier periods gave way to a joyful affirmation of the quiet life in a humble world praising its Creator.

If the tendency of preceding representations had been to spiritualize the concrete furnishings of the world, the iconographic interest now reversed itself. The growing realism expressed itself in a naïve curiosity about the material "technique" of the sacred mystery. The artist, we may say, tried to answer visually the frightened question of the Virgin, "Quo modo fiet istud? . . ." (Luke 1:34). The angel in the text of the Gospel answered: "The Holy Ghost shall come upon you and the Power of the Highest shall overshadow you. . . . For with God nothing shall be impossible." The union between the Creator and His creature is a mystery that cannot and need not be further explained in words;[23] in this way believers have accepted the doctrine. But the artist faces the task of making visible what the believer understands in a mystical nonphysical sense. He asks, "Quo modo?" "In what way?" God is the Father of Jesus through the medium of the Holy Ghost, both of them, of course, nonmaterial. The Holy Ghost was represented very early by the symbol of the Dove hovering over the head of the Virgin or near the Archangel. When God Himself was added to the representation, He was shown as a bearded old man with the papal triple crown on His head as the sign of His supreme authority. But the answer to the question "Quo modo?" demanded more. Therefore a semiphysical connection between God and the Virgin was indicated by a band of rays emanating from the mouth of God and aimed at the womb, the heart, or the right ear of Mary. Augustine had already pondered about the mode of impregnation. The biblical text says that "recipies in utero" (as Jerome translated the Greek words "en gastri syllempse"). Augustine mitigated the reference to a bodily organ by speaking about the "uterus cordis," the womb of the heart, which was reached through the ear by the obedient acceptance of the divine message (impregnatio per aurem).[24] Therefore the Annunciation and the hierogamy are really the same event, and the words of the Archangel, "Ave gratia plena," and Mary's answer, "Ecce ancilla Domini" are not words spoken about the event; they are the event itself. They appear in some pictures as banderols, either held by the two persons or coming as written letters out of their mouths. In Jan van Eyck's *Annunciation* in the Washington National Gallery, the answer of the Virgin is written from right to left, thus indicating its origin and direction; on the Ghent Altarpiece the words of Mary are written upside down, so that "ecce" is nearest to her lips.

Often the Dove of the Holy Ghost or a minute infant shouldering a cross float down on the rays coming from the mouth of God, thus uniting the three Persons of the Trinity with Mary. But this iconographic variation was indignantly rejected as "reprehensible" by Antonius of Florence (1389–1459) because it would deny the incarnation of Christ "ex substantia Virginis," in contradiction to the Athanasian credal formula: "Begotten, not made";[25] in the eighteenth century it was finally condemned as heretical by Benedict XIV.

A still cruder materialization of the concept of the paternity of God can be seen in some examples in which God is represented as blowing the Holy Ghost into the ear of Mary with a kind of tube or blowpipe (e.g., relief in the tympanum of the Dome of Wurzburg, ca. 1430–1450). Another case of this strange mixture of mysticism and technical realism is found in Crivelli's *Annunciation with St. Emidius* (1486). He follows the convention of representing the mystery of the Incarnation by a bundle of golden rays coming from Heaven to the Virgin, who is seated in a small room inside a Renaissance palazzo; but in order to make the passage of the rays from the outside to the inside visually plausible, he breaks the ornamental frieze of the building with a special little half-round window, thus reconciling the supreme power of the Almighty with the optical experience of profane life.

As Christian myths and legends spread, they encountered everywhere folk tales, sagas, and rituals of pre-Christian origin. These were either rejected as superstitions or reinterpreted in Christian terms. (The word "mythos" acquired its meaning of untruth only through the polemical writings of the Church Fathers against pagan beliefs.) Reinterpretation was required when such concepts had found literary form in the books of classical authorities. Examples of such syncretistic efforts were the encyclopedic works of Isidore of Seville (560–636) and the many "Bestiaries" which, throughout the Middle Ages, formed the basis for all animal symbolism in the visual arts. Such reconciliations between the scholarship of classical antiquity and the teachings of the Christian Church were occasionally quaint and artificial, but they were theologically acceptable as long as they did not contradict the authority of Holy Scripture and orthodox doctrine. However, a very different situation was created when non-Christian legendary motifs were superimposed upon traditional Christian teachings in such a way that the meaning of the religious message was essentially changed. This happened at the end of the Middle Ages. In the iconography of the Annunciation this final stage of allegoristic expansion was reached when the mystery of the Incarnation was interwoven with the colorful secular imagery of the Unicorn legend. This fable, of problematic origin,[26] was known in many variations from the Far East to the Mediterranean region. It had been incorporated into the vocabulary of the Vulgate when Jerome chose the word "Unicorn" to translate an obscure Hebrew term that appeared seven times in different books of the Old Testament, indicating a fabulous monster of invincible power. As the mightiest of all animals, it was used as a symbol of Christ. Similarly, the familiar story of the Unicorn saving all other animals by dipping its horn into water poisoned by serpents could be interpreted as an allegory of Christ saving mankind from the poison of the devil. But the catching of the Unicorn by luring it into the lap of a virgin, a story that, with its transparent sexual symbols, appealed very much to the taste of medieval court society, was a different matter. There exist quite a number of illustrations from the fifteenth and sixteenth centuries in which the Annunciation is presented as the Hunt of the Unicorn. The Virgin sits in a garden surrounded by a wall, the traditional hortus conclusus of Canticles (4:12) with a covered well (Cant. 14:12), an ivory tower (Cant. 7:5), and a locked portal (Ezek. 44:2). She fondles the unicorn in her lap while outside the Archangel Gabriel, dressed as a hunter, blows his horn; the banderol coming from the horn shows the words of the angelic salutation. Gabriel holds on a leash three or four yelping dogs, their names written into the picture as "Veritas," "Justitia," "Pax," and "Misericordia." From afar the half figure of God blesses the rather incongruent scene.

In such explicit form, the unicorn iconogram was apparently never used for altarpieces, but as illustrations of books accessible only to a wealthy and sophisticated elite. Again, the Council of Trent in 1565 prohibited the continuation of the symbolistic game. The idea that God, the Virgin, and the Archangel Gabriel outwit the Unicorn Jesus so that the Incarnation could come about, that the dogs with the names of Christian virtues hound the Unicorn Christ to his virginal mother, that he is to be killed by the spear of the Archangel—all these ideas make little sense, either from a religious or a logical point of view.

It seems that in this bizarre representation the symbols and allegories of two totally unrelated myths had freed themselves from their original meanings and had joined together, not because they conveyed a common meaning, but because they were suggestive images of two unrelated concepts that could not be expressed without symbolization—visualizations of mysterious entities that in their essence remained invisible. For the nervous sensitivity and sensuality of late medieval high society, consistently fed and overfed on half-revealing, half-concealing symbolic references, a society devoted to masquerades, charades, and allegorical erotic games,[27] these riddles had no solutions and could therefore substitute for each other. By analogy to surrealism, the art style of a society overfed and fed up with realities, I propose to call this last phase of iconography "sursymbolism." What had happened was the triumph of content over meaning, an emphasis on the symbol for the symbol's own sake. After this last phase of Christian iconography, an obligatory canon for the representation of the Annunciation was no longer possible.

NOTES

1. E. Panofsky, *Studies in iconology*. New York, 1939; *Meaning in the visual arts*. Garden City, N.Y., 1955. G. Hemerén, "Representation and meaning in the visual arts. A study in the methodology of iconography and iconology." *Lund Studies in Philosophy*, I. Lund, 1969. J. Bialostocki, "Iconography." In P. Wiener (Ed.), *Dictionary of the history of ideas*. New York, 1973. M. Schapiro, *Words and pictures*. The Hague, 1973.

2. R. Palmer, *Hermeneutics*. Evanston, Ill., 1969. H. Gadamer, *Wahrheit und Methode*. Tübingen, 1960. O. F. Bollnow, *Das Verstehen*. München, 1949.

3. H. A. Wolfson, *Philosophy of the Church Fathers*. Cambridge, Mass., 1956.

4. M. S. Torry, *Bible hermeneutics*. New York, 1890. Chap. 3. G. Ebeling, "Hermeneutics." In *Religion in Geschichte und Gegenwart* (3. Aufl.), 1959. Vol. 3, pp. 242–262.

Wolfgang
M. Zucker

5. J. Daniélou, *Origen*. Paris, 1948. H. v. Balthasar, *Origines, Geist und Form*. Salzburg, 1938.

6. M. Foucault, *The order of things. An archeology of the human sciences*. New York, 1971. Chaps. 2 and 3.

7. J. Daniélou, *Sacramentum futuri. Études sur les origines de la typologie biblique*. Paris, 1950. L. Réau, *Iconographie de l'art chrétien*. Paris, 1953. Vol. 1, pp. 192ff.

8. H. Rahner, *Griechische Mythen in Christlicher Deutung*. Zurich, 1957.

9. H. Cornell, *Biblia Pauperum*. Stockholm, 1925.

10. *The Golden Legend of Jacobus de Voragine* (G. Ryan and H. Ripperger, trans.). London, 1941.

11. E. Male, *The Gothic image. Religious art in France of the thirteenth century*. New York, 1958. Pp. 390ff. (Originally published, 1913.)

12. D. M. Robb, "The iconography of the Annunciation in the fourteenth and fifteenth centuries." *Art Bulletin* 18 (1936). L. Rudrauf, *L'Annunciation*. Paris, 1943. M. E. Gössmann, *Die Verkündigung an Maria im dogmatischen Verständnis des Mittelalters*. München, 1957. L. Réau, loc. cit., Vol. 1, pp. 174–194. G. Schiller, *Ikonographie der Christlichen Kunst*. (2. Aufl.). Gütersloh, 1969. Vol. 1, pp. 44–65. J. J. Mak, *Middleeuwse Kerst-Voorstellingen*. Utrecht-Brussel, 1948.

13. E. Hennecker and W. Scheemelcher, *New Testament Apocrypha*. Philadelphia, 1965. Vol. 1, pp. 368ff.

14. Ibid., pp. 405ff.

15. Molanus. *De historia sanctarum imaginum et picturarum*. Louvain, 1771.

16. H. Rahner, *Symbole der Kirche*. Salzburg, 1964. Pp. 91–176.

17. E. Panofsky, "The Friedsam Annunciation and the problem of the Ghent Altarpiece." *Art Bulletin* 17 (1935).

18. Y. Hirn, *The sacred shrine*. London, 1912. Pp. 281ff.

19. H. Rahner, "Flumina de Ventre Christi. Die Patristische Auslegung von Joh 7:37–38." In *Symbole der Kirche*. Salzburg, 1964. Pp. 177ff.

20. J. Schafer, *Das Handbuch der Malerei vom Berge Athos aus dem handschriftlichen, neugriechischen Urtext übertragen*. Trier, 1885.

21. Cf. note 17.

22. E. Panofsky, *Early Netherlandish painting*. Cambridge, Mass., 1958. Pp. 30ff.

23. R. Pieper, "Die Auslegung der Worte Spiritus Sanctus superveniet". . . . In *Theologie und Glaube*, 1913. Bd. 5, pp. 751ff.

24. S. Augustinus. Sermon CXCVI. In Natale Domini XIII. Migne S. L. 38.

25. Quoted by Robb, loc. cit., p. 256.

26. O. Shepard, *The lore of the unicorn*. New York, 1967. Chap. 2. (Originally published, 1913.)

27. J. Huizinga, *The waning of the Middle Ages*. New York, 1949. Chaps. 8, 12, 15, 17.

Walter Hess

Formal Analysis of a Painting by Jan Vermeer

As a storyteller Jan Vermeer may be called a "minimalist" among the painters of cultured middle-class interiors. He is satisfied with showing a corner of a room, the limits of which remain undetermined in three directions (see illustration). Of the event represented in the painting he shows no more than what a casual passer-by could gather at a glance. For a brief moment he reveals the intimate sphere of two persons who believe themselves to be unobserved and about whom the secret onlooker is given no further information. The lady is about to sip the last drop from her glass, the gentleman holds on to the pitcher, from which he probably poured wine for her and perhaps is about to pour again. The woman, as Vermeer's contemporaries would have known, is a courtesan. Thus the painting belongs to the gallantry genre, whose customary attributes were wine and musical instruments.

Vermeer is the only Dutch painter in this category whom modern artists, from the impressionists to the abstract constructivists, have acknowledged as being far above the others and congenial to the modern spirit. He appealed to the impressionists by the unliterary purity of his vision and by the lucidity of his colors, which appear as light or, to put it the other way round, by a kind of light that combines the colors of objects in sonorous chords without allowing anything to be submerged in darkness. Every element of the work has a share in the orchestration of the color theme but the concrete reality of the objects is

Translated from the German by Rudolf Arnheim.
  The following attempt at interpretation of a painting was carried out with students in a seminar of the Staatliche Hochschule für bildende Künste in West Berlin. One of the bases for this work was Rudolf Arnheim's research on the theory of perception.

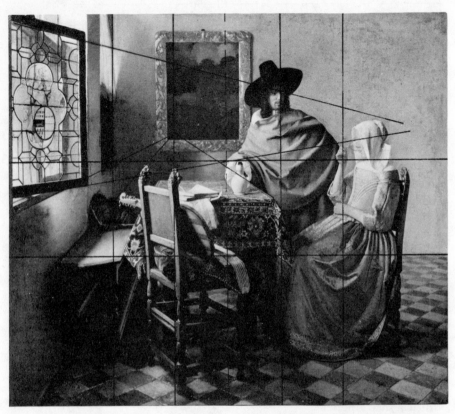

1 Jan Vermeer, *Girl Drinking with a Gentleman*. Courtesy Staatliche
Museen Preussischer Kulturbesitz Gemäldegalerie Berlin (West).

nevertheless preserved. Although the subject matter defines the picture as segmentary in space and momentary in time, the work is wholly unified and complete in a pictorial sense. It reposes in the equilibrium of the objects constituting it, whether one views them as volumes in space or as surface areas within the organized picture plane.

The two-dimensional order discloses relations that are simple but complex at the same time. Horizontally the area of the picture can be divided according to the ratio of the golden section by a vertical connecting the left outline of the woman's skirt with the right edge of the table cover and continuing as the central axis of the male figure, which is accented by the breaks in the folds of his cape. When the same ratio is applied to the other side of the picture, a second vertical divides the total width along the forward edge of the chair and crosses one of the finials on its back exactly at the tip. Thus the two axes determining the composition so fundamentally are found to articulate the picture according to the same, eminently harmonious proportion.

The central area, delimited by the two verticals, is dominated by the man's grasp of the pitcher. The axis of that pitcher conforms to a further vertical located very close to the central axis of the total canvas and sustained underneath by the right frontal leg of the chair and above by the inside edge of the golden picture frame on the wall. Thus the two human figures are located in the right half of the painting, although it may be noted that if one were to reduce the total area of Vermeer's canvas to a square by trimming it on the right, the woman's back would still be included in it.

One can go farther and apply the golden ratio again, namely to the major component of one of the subdivisions described a moment ago, i.e., the distance between the right finial of the chair and the right border of the canvas. In that way one can obtain an additional vertical, which crosses the foot of the wine glass. The distance between this new vertical and the right border of the canvas is exactly equal to the width of the central zone between the two primary axes and also to the distance between the left border of the canvas and the right limit of the more remote, closed window with the blue curtain. This same vertical coincides with the right leg of the bench.

Finally, the golden section can be applied to the vertical dimension of the painting as well. This division produces a horizontal line running at the height of the woman's wrist and touching the top of the pitcher.

Walter
Hess

171

Observations of this kind determine some factors of what might be called a pictorial planimetry, which creates a harmonious balance of shapes, comparable to the relations of hues within color chords. However, these formal devices do not impose themselves on the beholder as conspicuously intentional.

When the planimetric order is examined in its relation to the structure of the three-dimensional picture space in the depth dimension, one notices tension as well as compensation. Vermeer constructs his central perspective for a station point close by, which makes for strong foreshortening, tangible nearness of the foreground objects, and rapid recession from front to back. The viewer is closest to the open window. If the bottom edge of that window is continued through the picture, the line will be seen to cross the right finial of the chair and to touch the top of the pitcher and the foot of the wine glass—three spots we found to be instrumental in the establishment of the proportional subdivision of the picture plane.

The vanishing point for the orthogonal edges of the room lies on one of the principal verticals, which crosses the right finial of the chair. That perspective center is located close to the lower left corner of the painting on the wall. The vanishing point establishes the eye level of the viewer and makes him look into the room from a height corresponding to the seated woman's forehead. Accordingly, we look up to the man as a towering figure. The perspective also defines the station point of the observer and places him directly opposite the right edge of the chair, which comes so close. As we enter the room at this point and traverse its rapidly converging depth, our advance is arrested by the painting on the wall. From the quiet expanse of the painting, a perceptual gradient and a color crescendo lead downward to the woman, in accordance with the direction of the man's glance.

Along with the oblique lines of the window, the light enters and floods the room; it meets the woman head on and heightens the red-orange color of her dress to a maximum of intensity. The stained glass of the window acts as an overture to the unity of light and color, even though here the light is still predominant in shades of lemon yellow and orange. But red and blue are touched upon as well, and there are also the gradations of green, which pervade the color scheme of the entire painting as a supporting base.

Following the light, the viewer's glance descends from the left toward the middle ground but rises also on the wings of the perspective to the background, ascends to the golden frame of the painting, and advances again forward and downward to the seated woman. On our approach to the depth of the picture, however, we run into the backs of the chair and the musical instrument, which form an obstacle blocking off the middle ground. In fact, we are deflected and slide along the neck of the instrument and through a sequence of blues toward the corner of the room and upward to the blue transparency of the curtain.

Since, however, the chair and the musical instrument turn their backs to us, they look toward the middle ground and direct us inward and upward again to the central group. That group, perceived in three-dimensional space, rises on a quadrilateral ground plan as a configuration of obliquely oriented parallels, the nearest corner being represented by the protruding leg of the chair, the farthest by the male figure. We note that these two corners of the three-dimensional order are located on two principal verticals of the proportional subdivision in the two-dimensional order.

Vermeer's composition conforms fully to the psychological observation according to which the viewer identifies normally with the left side of a picture and proceeds toward the right, from the zone of primary attention to a zone of more efficient vision. All perceptual paths come to rest in the seated figure. However, at the same time they overlay one another in such a way that, when viewed in simultaneity, they constitute a perfectly balanced, highly complex structure.

It is hardly possible to capture in words the total structure created and the substance and meaning conveyed by the formal devices that have been enumerated here so incompletely. Ludwig Goldscheider, in his monograph on Jan Vermeer, has tried to express it metaphorically by suggesting that this painter takes hold of a single moment the way one seizes upon a thought that cannot be fathomed by any reflection and in whose light the world is seen as though for the first time, new and untouched. The art historian Kurt Badt has spoken in his *Kunsttheoretische Versuche* of "the mysterious power of a view of reality that here makes its heightened and lasting appearance." "Existences rather than moments" attain presence in our perception.[1]

Walter
Hess

NOTES   1. After the completion of this paper, the author came across a study by the Russian art historian Michail Alpatow, "Die *Strasse in Delft von Jan Vermeer," Studien zur Geschichte der westeuropäischen Kunst.* Moscow, 1939 and 1963, German translation, Cologne, 1974. Alpatow's analysis of proportionality in Vermeer's paintings arrives at analogous results.

Dore Ashton

Art and Social Change

Some years ago when I was in Rome, I met an archeological student who announced that he alone knew of a certain place secreting the remains of an ancient Roman culture. We packed a picnic lunch, took some ridiculously rudimentary tools, and off we went to the rolling hills. We started digging at once on a lovely summer's day, and within minutes I had unearthed a terra-cotta foot. Next came a chin, then a forehead. We began to dig furiously and the sherds were coming fast. Suddenly it occurred to me that there was an unusual number of historical remains in a single place, and I looked carefully at the foot: it was without doubt mass-produced. What we had found, I feel sure, was a factory dump of ancient days. Discards. Multiples. This thought changed my whole feeling for the admittedly elegant arch and beautiful toes of my fragmentary foot. Had I been a sociologist, I would have been pleased to speculate on the kind of culture that had factories for producing sculpture. Had I been a pure aesthete, I would have thrown away my vulgar finds. Being neither, I have always had an ambivalent feeling about this emblem of a mysterious past.

It is almost too obvious to begin with the truism that art *is* change in its essence. All the history of art is studded with evidence that the nature of art is to change. Even those seemingly changeless cultures we are told about, where the same general forms are used again and again—certain so-called primitive cultures—can be seen in this light. I have never seen two identical African masks. To insist that change in art is rigidly aligned with change in society is to exclude all the troubling contradictions in the history of the arts. We are on very marshy ground. Even Karl Marx was not quite sure how to approach the linkage of art with social change. Starting as he did from a theory of total historical process—a distancing technique which is indispensable for an ideologist—he could make a *general* assumption that 175 social change effected artistic changes. It is the *particular* which evaded him. He could risk assuming that a society starving to death would produce little art: "a sense confined within harsh necessity has only restricted sensibility" or, as Brecht so admirably summed it up: "Erst kommt das Fressen, dann kommt die Moral." But Marx had to admit that "In art, it is recognized that specific flourishing periods hardly conform to the general development of society, that is, of the material base, the skeleton, so to speak, which produces them." And Lenin echoed him: "The phenomenon is *richer* than the law." In short, neither of the great ideologists could quite account for the contradictions provided by the history of art. The law, as they saw it, was that there could be no pure, autonomous, "immanent" history, either for science or for art; yet they sensed, as we still do, that perhaps both the pure, immanent history and the history extended from social change were held in suspension in the arts. All subsequent Marxist interpreters of the arts have had to deal with the dilemma.

What invariably hinders the Marxist interpreter is the seeming independence of form—what Focillon called "The Life of Forms." A dialectical materialist is by definition wholly historical. Therefore a sensitive Marxist commentator such as Lukács must denounce what he calls the "idealistic de-historicizing of form" and the "idealistic inflation of form" which he says become most obvious in modern art's "transformation of forms into mystical and autonomous, even 'eternal' entities."

This is precisely the same basis on which Meyer Schapiro attacked Alfred Barr's catalogue, *Cubism and Abstract Art*, for the 1936 exhibition. Schapiro reproached Barr for presenting the history of modern art as "an eternal, immanent process among the artists." He attacked what he called "the pretension that art was above history through the creative energy or personality of the artist." And he pointed out with disapproval that new attitudes to the art of primitives, children, and madmen made it possible to cut across barriers of time and place. As an historical materialist, he could not accept the de-historicizing of forms.

Artists themselves have never been consistent in their view of their relationship to their time. Most artists accept that in the broadest sense they are "of their time." Matisse, speaking of imitators of old masters, said: "Such painters are of no value to anyone because, whether we want to or not, we belong to our time and we share its opinions, preferences, delusions. All artists bear the imprint of their time, but great artists are those in which this stamp is most deeply impressed. . . . Whether we want it or not, between our period and ourselves an indissoluble bond is established." He is echoed in the statements of countless modern painters. Yet most of them would agree with the poet Karl Shapiro that "It's true that a man is a product of his times, but mostly in unseen, unthought ways. A great artist may be affected more by a piece of furniture in his room than by wars raging all over the world. If I hadn't been vaccinated when I was five, maybe I would have died of smallpox; that makes me a twentieth-century man."

On the other hand, many artists have hated to be immured in a time or a place. Picasso says, "to me there is no past or future in art," and he probably would have withered Lukács with a witticism if Lukács had sneered at the idea of eternal entities. In some cases you would have to controvert evidence to insist that an artist be bound by some time or place. The British literary critic V. S. Pritchett has pointed out that "as men and women we inherit society and whether we approve or do not approve of our time, we assume we all belong. . . . But the artist, in searching for the identity of his irritant, may very well discover that he does not belong to our century. . . . Blake, born of the dying race of craftsmen, speaks clear across every movement of the nineteenth century to today. Stendhal is notorious for being a hundred years ahead of his time when he seemed out of date or irrelevant in his own."

Something in the work of art, then, resists surrendering to ideology, whether aesthetic or historical. A work of art is polyvalent. It can be seen as a document, as it is invariably seen by Marxists, or it can be seen as a transcendence, or as any number of other things. And, if you adopt enough distance, a work of art can be seen as either an avatar of social change or an effect of social change. There are always legitimate bases for such speculation. Probably the art historian Ludwig Goldscheider was right when he said that the past changes as rapidly as the present.

To see how rapidly the past changes, or, to put it in a different way, to see how consistent is the necessity for historical interpretation, we have only to look in various sectors of the history of art. Take the case of Courbet. For some he was the inventor of realism in painting, which meant nothing more than that he painted what he saw. For others, he was the first modern painter whose political stance was projected through his art. The Communist poet Louis Aragon looked for, and located, the political implications of Courbet's work. "The appearance of the

Dore
Ashton

177

Courbet phenomenon in painting," he said, "coincides with the awakening of the giant, the worker in that century, and Courbet might well owe this or that to preceding painters but the rupture, that is the *materialist* attitude, doesn't come from them but from the rising giant." Since Courbet was a confirmed political radical, and since Courbet's closest associates during his later years in Paris were political theorists of some note, Aragon's assertions cannot be disregarded. Nevertheless, there is a whole other history of Courbet, to which the British art historian Alan Bowness has addressed himself. I suspect that Bowness's undertaking is somewhat spurred by the current vogue for politicizing the history of art—a vogue which, like any other, has some unsavory implications.

Bowness, in a recently published study, concentrates on Courbet's earlier works which, along with all the rest, have been dealt with as though they were pure exemplifications of his political theories. To restore the balance, Bowness surveys the art of the period, notes that there were many artists dealing with similar themes—that is, rural life or provincial mores—and speculates on derivations other than exclusively political considerations. He notes that at the time Courbet was working on such canvases as the *Burial at Ornans*, the novels in Georges Sand's rural series were extremely popular. Sand herself, who had strong political interests, had made a point of saying that when these "country" novels were written, "I had no system, no revolutionary pretension in literature." It was quite in fashion to paint scenes of life in the provinces. Bowness adds that Courbet's closest association with an art critic in the mid- to late 1840s was with Champfleury, who specifically liked genre paintings that were "solid and not chic." If we add to these points the fact that Courbet's autobiographical statements had been visibly consistent, and that he more than once expressed the desire to paint whatever he could see, it seems likely that Courbet in his early years invested these scenes with little or no political significance. What Bowness does is to offer the other considerations in a painter's oeuvre, and to give a proper warning against oversimplification.

Efforts to gain distance and to see Impressionism as significant of social change have not always been successful, but when well-argued, the sociopolitical interpretation of Impressionism is important. Once again, Meyer Schapiro is perhaps the most lucid exponent of this approach. In 1937, he addressed himself to the moral aspect of Impressionism, seeing "in its discovery of a constantly changing phenomenal outdoor world of which the shapes depended on the momentary position of the casual or mobile spectator" an "implicit criticism of symbolic social and domestic formalities."

The Impressionists' preference for such motifs as picnics, promenades, and boating scenes—scenes of what Schapiro called "spontaneous sociability"—meant to Schapiro that the Impressionists were painting to a certain group in the social system—namely, the "urban promenader and the refined consumer of luxury goods." When, shortly after, the post-Impressionists arrived on the scene, they ushered in the era in the 1880s when the alienated artist first became visible. The new bourgeoisie and the extravagances of industrial capitalism could not support the increasingly private tendency in the arts. According to Schapiro, the artists "did not know the underlying economic and social causes of their own disorder and moral insecurity." The appearance of the mass culture caught them unprepared. Some, however, reacted as Seurat did: "Instead of rebelling against the moral consequences of capitalism, [he] attached himself like a contented engineer to its progressive technical side and accepted the popular forms of lower-class recreation and commercialized entertainment as the subjects of a monumentalized art." Schapiro summarizes his argument in these terms: "If the tendencies of the arts after Impressionism toward an extreme subjectivism and abstraction are already evident in Impressionism, it is because the isolation of the individual and of the higher forms of culture from the older social supports, the renewed ideological opposition of mind and nature, individual and society, proceed from social and economic causes which had already existed before Impressionism."

Schapiro could marshal some support for his arguments from the artists themselves. Pissarro, a socialist, called Impressionist art "absolutely social, anti-authoritarian, and anti-mystical." But perhaps we might say the same of Degas' works, knowing that Degas was a political reactionary of the most unappealing kind. As for the post-Impressionists, it happens that Seurat, Signac, Cross, and the critic Fénéon were quite seriously committed to a kind of anarcho-socialist point of view. When they came to discuss their art, however, there was rarely an allusion to sociopolitical terms of assessment. Signac did, in 1891, attempt to make an argument that the neo-Impressionists were political artists. He spoke of the picturesque studies of workers' housing at Saint-Ouen or Montrouge, of blacksmiths and workers, as indicative of their political interests. He said that the "pleasures of decadence: balls, kick-choruses, circuses such as that of the painter Seurat, who had such a lively feeling for the degradation of our era of transition, bear witness to the great social struggle that is now taking place between workers and capitalism." Yet he also insisted that the paintings of neo-Impressionism result "from a purely aesthetic emotion produced by the pictorial quality of things and beings," and that they "contain that unconscious social quality with which contemporary literature is already marked." Not even so fiery a radical as Signac, who was still forcefully demanding the commitments of fellow artists in 1935 at the great congress of left-wing intellectuals in Paris, could bring himself to see the greatness of Seurat as lying purely in Seurat's observation of the "decadence" of his capitalist era.

If we accept the polyvalence of works of art, we can accept even the idea that the same artist can be at once political and formal, or informal and committed, or topical and abstract, depending on circumstances. During the 1930s, Stuart Davis serenely painted "formalist" pictures while taking the lead in vigorous social actions. Others occasionally produced socially meaningful—as it was called—art, and still others produced *only* topical or political works.

Even within the oeuvre of a single artist, the several attitudes toward history, aesthetics, and social change can be interchanged, probably without ever quite finding the correct approach. (Only vulgar Marxists suppose a "correct" approach anyway.) Take two paintings of de Kooning of the same period. One is an abstraction: a canvas swept over with forces, in which the initial thought is stated ambiguously, in which the image— the relationship of colors and forms—emerges with an emotional value that defies the word. It also defies analysis in terms of history or social change unless we are to move far, far away and to speak from the bridgehead of total historical process. Perhaps from that remote outpost of dialectical logic, de Kooning's abstraction could be interpreted as the work of the artist alienated from capitalist society. More likely, however, such an image could better be contemplated from within the "immanent" history of modern art.

On the other hand, the painting called *Marilyn Monroe*, still swept on with expressionist élan, still showing the particular forms and colors peculiar to de Kooning, offers other possibilities. Here, perhaps, the painting can also be seen as a document bespeaking societal changes. The argument runs:

de Kooning takes a popular figure, whose renown has been spread around the world by the mass media. He stresses, in the caricatural mouth, the imagery of the masses which derives from newspapers, cigarette and automobile advertisements on highways, and popular magazines. The painting, then, is an oblique commentary on the changing social image. Yet, if we see the painting *within* de Kooning's total oeuvre to date, we would have to adjust our approach to allow for the inner coherence of his formal style which, I think, partakes of another kind of history.

Another example: Philip Guston, around the same time de Kooning painted his abstraction, also painted an abstraction. His painting, naturally, differs from de Kooning's, although the two share certain artistic assumptions. Guston's forms cleave to different spaces and tend to vibrate in place. His colors stay closer in tonality. His brushwork, while spontaneous and immediate, tends to stress the cohesiveness of his small units within a space that could be interpreted as infinite. In the light of the immanent history of modern painting, Guston's abstraction partakes of a period style, certainly, but does it stand for social change?

On the other hand, some years later, Guston renounces abstraction and determines, consciously, to paint subjects that relate to his experience in a turbulent political century. Specifically, he refers to the holocaust, and indirectly he refers to all political repression everywhere. These paintings are at once topical and what Lukács would ironically call eternal. They can just as easily be related to the torture scenes in early Renaissance paintings as they can to Goya or to the social realism of the 1930s.

Like Guston, the sculptor David Smith had had strong social impulses in the 1930s. Among his early works were several referring directly to the horrors of the Nazi period, and several others describing the plight of the American worker during the Depression. Even when he embarked on his abstractions, he retained references in the titles to his concern with the workingman. Yet Smith's later abstract sculptures would have to be seen within the immanent history of modern sculpture to be comprehensible even historically. He never lost his desire to share in the radical social currents of his time, and when he worked in Voltri, a small Italian town with a socialist mayor, he took special pleasure in the concourse with workingmen, and even wondered whether he wasn't working better because of

Dore
Ashton

181

the ministrations of the socialist mini-society in which he temporarily found himself.

In the long view, again, Smith's gigantic sculptures (he said he wanted to make a sculpture as large as a locomotive) reflect the giant industrial society. But then, in completely different terms, we would say that the other sculptor, Tony Smith, also does this. Tony Smith's austere, monumental sculptures, scaled to public places, and commensurate with urban architecture, *feel* as though they belong to a specific time and place. Still others leave us with no doubt. The work of the sculptor Ed Kienholz is always specific. He tells us the time, he tells us the place. In fact, he re-enacts certain experiences that are immediately hooked into place in American history. Despite occasional gestures toward a less limited interpretation, such as substituting clocks for faces on his effigies, Kienholz's work is basically topical, and intentionally so. The sculpture of Claes Oldenburg is often aimed at specific places, and always refers to the social situation in one way or another. But Oldenburg can be seen within a modern art tradition of anti-art, so that once again, only the longest perspective of the historical materialist can make the correct generality.

There are areas in modern art, however, in which the relationships to social changes are far more easy to discern. Long ago in modern art history the distinction between *homo faber*— he who makes something—and he who consumes began to be blurred. The "modern" man was the man who existed in a society radically altered by technological progress. A painting by Manet such as the vision of wistful girls at the railroad tracks could be—and *is* very often—interpreted as the product of a technologically-oriented society.

The possibility of enlargements—whether psychological or technical—did affect artists. Wagner's idea of the *Gesamtkunstwerk* was not solely an aesthetic effect of a great synthesizing creator. His interest in *spectacle* was abetted by the newly created means of dissemination. Publicity was Wagner's ally in the founding of the Bayreuth spectacles, and Nietzsche, his erstwhile admirer, smelled a rat. In fact, Nietzsche's rants against modernism were based on his sensitive reactions to the new element of spectacle in all the arts. As a believer in the redemptive value of the creative act, he sensed the threat when art was propelled out of its aesthetic precincts into the arena of historical life. For modern counterfeiting in the arts, he said, "the artist first seeks a less artistic public which loves uncondition-

Artifact

ally." Then, "he harangues the obscure instincts of the dissatisfied, ambitious, self-disguised spirits in a democratic age. Then one transfers the procedures of one art to the other arts, confounds the objectives of art with those of knowledge or the church or racial interests (nationalism) or philosophy—one pulls all the stops at once and awakens the dark suspicion that one may be a god."

Nietzsche's remarks on modern painters are particularly suggestive: "All these moderns are poets who wanted to be painters. One looks for dramas in history, another scenes of manners, this one translates religions, that one philosophies.. . . No one is simply a painter; all are archeologists, psychologists, theatrical producers of this or that recollection or theory. They enjoy our erudition, our philosophy. Like us, they are full and overfull of general ideas. They like a form not for the sake of what it is, but for the sake of what it expresses. They are sons of a scholarly, tormented and reflective generation—a thousand miles removed from the old masters who did not read and only thought of feasting their eyes."

Our sons of a scholarly, tormented, and reflective generation have most certainly availed themselves of the media, and have also deliberately sought to dismantle the arts, using a battery of tools derived from scholars. The dismantling often takes on a theatrical aura, as Nietzsche observed. When Richard Huelsenbeck led the first revolutionary generation of artists in the Dada spectacles at the end of World War I, the "staging" of spectacles was very important. At its most blatant, the attack on art occurs *only* in spectacles, such as those performed by the so-called Destructivist movement. (Here it is of some ironic significance that in a well-publicized Destructivist event, in which the assassination of some live chickens called down the wrath of animal lovers, one of the prime movers was a man called Harvey Matusow. This Matusow had once gained notoriety in a very different spectacle when, during the McCarthy hearings, he was a key informer.)

The pressure to act upon society, in the name of art, has been mounting ever since Nietzsche's time. The actors in this drama most often assume an ideological position. They are specifically directing their "events" against the capitalist, or the bourgeois mentality, at least in the West. They associate the work of art with the possessiveness of the privileged classes and, in removing the possibility of a permanent, possessable object, they deprive society of its cherished status symbols. More deeply, they

Dore
Ashton

183

reflect the vacuum produced when, as Nietzsche once again put it, Western society discovered that God is dead. Into this vacuum moves the spiritual energy of the artist who assumes the role, not of maker, but of director of ethics.

During the past fifteen years, there have been numerous attempts to de-emphasize the work of art as an object and to "ethicize" the world through the performance of the artist. These have ranged from earlier Happenings by Allan Kaprow, in which there is a distinct theatrical, aesthetic increment, to recent works by Hans Haacke, in which the aesthetic is programmatically rejected, and in which a distinct political gesture is intended. (The exhibition rejected by the Guggenheim Museum contained photographs and statistics about tenements in New York and their unprincipled owners.)

The most startling recent theatrical phenomena, however, can be credited to the German artist, Joseph Beuys. Like his countryman Huelsenbeck, Beuys sees the function of the artist as the creator of a new kind of man, a man with liberated senses, released from the unfreedoms imposed by the rigidity of technological societies, and no longer bound by the idea that art is dependent on craft. Beuys borrows liberally from all the disciplines and fulfills quite neatly Nietzsche's description of the "modern" artist: he is more critic than artist. Although Beuys's elemental themes are closer to Nietzsche than to twentieth-century materialism, and although he sees the capitalist dependence on technology as an evil (he uses a great deal of Christian terminology), he is dependent on "the media," technology's largest contribution to our society, for the dissemination of his views. The photographs of his ascetic, sometimes secretly smiling face, of his hallmark, the gray felt hat, of his performing various rites are indispensable to his functioning. Moreover, he has frequently been recorded and taped for television and seems never to perform a solitary act. His stance as *agent provocateur* within a very special system—that of *Wirtschaftswunder* Germany—has been effective. The whole intellectual world was engaged in his struggle with the Academy, and the Academy, in this instance, is merely a symbolic institution standing for the broadest general political situation within Germany.

Beuys's chief intent is apparently to found a new sociology based on the polarity of reason and emotion. "Freedom," he says, "is the ability of the individual to bring into being new causes." And these causes, it would appear, are never to be born if we continue to honor what he calls "man's stubborn rationalism." In order to disturb the rationalist patterns he, the artist personified, must take to the arena. He must remove the old aesthetic distance. The only means is spectacle which, as in the days of Wagner, is cloaked in an aura of pagan rite. The shamanism apparent in Beuys's "actions" is emphasized by the mysteries of his "scores"—those written notations with fragments of theological, philosophical, and aesthetic terminology that both exclude and mystify his adherents and suggest that he is the keeper of essential mysteries. When he then moves into the political arena, maintaining that he who functions both as artist and as work of art will effect change, he substitutes for the charisma of the traditional political leader the charisma of the shaman. Here, art and social change are in mortal conflict.

Beuys works in so-called democratic Germany, and undeniably his background as a fighter in World War II has tinctured his thought. Many artists are working in countries in which political systems were radically altered after that war. In many cases they pursue the same tendencies as Western democratic countries, perhaps for similar reasons. The whole movement into "conceptual" art, in which philosophical speculation supersedes the object, has found fertile territory in Eastern Europe. The Aesopian character of much post-World War II art can be discerned throughout the world. In Czechoslovakia, for example, Jiri Kolar developed his poetic sublanguage in which many motifs could be hidden, but not ultimately. Few could decipher his eruptions of words, or even some of his imagery. All the same, into the documentation comes allusion. A work called "Hair," which is a seemingly innocent surrealist composition, emerges nonetheless as a memento of Auschwitz. In his biographical notes, it is recorded that during certain periods of the Stalinist regime in Czechoslovakia, he could not publish his poetry and turned instead to making collages of fragments of words and visual symbols. All of his work is turned away from overt meaning, carries hidden innuendoes, and develops in an esoteric tradition specifically linked to politically repressive conditions. Here art and social change are indissolubly linked, but the artist moves, perhaps as he has always moved, to free himself from the restrictions imposed by this or that society and system. Nowhere is it more clear than in the work of an artist such as Kolar that a work of art is always both a social fact and an aesthetic fact. If, in some century to come, young archeologists were pondering the remains of a Beuys or a Kolar, in the case of Beuys they would be confronted with texts and pictorial documents of events, which

Dore
Ashton

185

would undoubtedly be classified as original sociological sources. In the case of Kolar, there might be texts or commentary, but the works themselves would have to be read independently as well.

Mary Henle, professor of psychology on the Graduate Faculty of the New School for Social Research, is a well-known figure in the scholarly world of psychology. Her numerous publications attest to the range of her professional inquiry, extending in the present volume to the frontier between psychology and art. A contributor to leading journals, she is the editor of *Documents of Gestalt Psychology* and *Selected Papers of Wolfgang Köhler,* as well as *Historical Conceptions of Psychology,* which she coedited with Julian Jaynes and John J. Sullivan (Springer: 1973).